Managing Outcomes through Collaborative Care

The Application of CareMapping and Case Management

The Center for Case Management
Karen Zander, Editor

AHA books are published by American Hospital Publishing, Inc., an American Hospital Association company

Library of Congress Cataloging-in-Publication Data

Managing outcomes through collaborative care : the application of
   CareMapping and case management / The Center for Case Management ;
   Karen Zander, editor.
         p.   cm.
      Includes bibliographical references (p.   ).
      ISBN 1-55648-132-2
      1. Hospitals–Case management services.   2. Medical protocols.
   3. Medical records.   I. Zander, Karen S., 1948-   .
   RA975.5.C36M36   1995
   362.1'1'068–dc20   94-47919
                                                                                           CIP

Catalog no. 027103

Printed in the USA

AHA is a service mark of the American Hospital Association used under license by American Hospital Publishing, Inc.

Text set in Century Textbook
4M–03/95–0397

Audrey Kaufman, Senior Editor
Nancy Charpentier, Editor
Peggy DuMais, Production Coordinator
Luke Smith, Cover Designer
Marcia Bottoms, Executive Editor
Brian Schenk, Books Division Director

Contents

List of Figures v

About the Editor viii

Contributors ix

Preface xi

Acknowledgments xiii

Chapter 1. Collaborative Care: Two Effective Strategies
            for Positive Outcomes 1
            Karen Zander

Chapter 2. The Physician's New Agenda 39
            John Kleinman, MD

Chapter 3. Program Design 59
            Karen Zander

Chapter 4. CareMap Project Management 95
            Susan P. Kyzer

Chapter 5. CareMap Development and Implementation 115
            Kathleen M. Andolina

Chapter 6. The Uses of Variance 131
            Patricia Potter

Chapter 7. Integration of CareMap Tools into the Documentation
            System 149
            Maria Hill

Chapter 8. Case Management Designed for the Care Continuum 165
            Kathleen Bower, DNSc

Chapter 9. Program Evaluation 177
            Mary Crabtree Tonges and Judith L. Brett, PhD

Chapter 10. A Look to the Future 195
            Karen Zander

List of Figures

Figure 1-1. Evolution of Trends toward Collaborative Care 3

Figure 1-2. Case Type as Common Denominator 5

Figure 1-3. Case Management Plan Excerpt: Scoliosis 8

Figure 1-4. Excerpts from Time Line Overview:
Uncomplicated MI (DRG 122) 10

Figure 1-5. Critical Path and Variance Record: Myocardial Infarction 12

Figure 1-6. CareMap Tool Grid: Congestive Heart Failure 16

Figure 1-7. The CareMap Formula 18

Figure 1-8. Problem/Outcome Index + Critical Path = CareMap Tool 18

Figure 1-9. Case Management Ground Rules 21

Figure 1-10. Case Management Rationale 23

Figure 1-11. Recommended Percentages of Patients Covered by CareMap
Tools, Care Management, and Case Management 23

Figure 1-12. Expanding Scope of Accountability 24

Figure 1-13. Effects of CareMap Systems and Collaborative Care
on Physician Practice 32

Figure 1-14. Comparison of Generic Steps in Clinical Decision Making 34

Figure 2-1. Hypothetical Relations between Health Benefits and Cost
of Care as Useful Additions Are Made to Care 43

Figure 2-2. Levels at Which Quality May Be Assessed 45

Figure 2-3. Cycle of Outcome-Based Care 47

Figure 2-4. CQI Tenets in the Cycle of Outcome-Based Care 47

Figure 2-5. MCCAP Model for Quality of Care Evaluation and Improvement . . 52

Figure 3-1. Flowchart: From CQI to Ownership by Operations 62

Figure 3-2. Progression of Education for Outcome-Based Practice 64

Figure 3-3. Recommended Infrastructure for Implementation
and Maintenance of a Collaborative Care Program 66

Figure 3-4. The Cog's Ladder Model of Group Development 67

Figure 3-5. Levels of Teams in a Collaborative Care Program 68

Figure 3-6. Case Type Collaborative Care Team: Development Plan
following CareMap Tool Authoring 69

Figure 3-7. Health One Mercy Hospital — CABG 71

Figure 3-8. Newton-Wellesley Hospital Collaborative Care
Group Practice Members 73

Figure 3-9. NWH Collaborative Care Project Manager:
Summary of Major Areas of Performance 74

Figure 3-10. Forms Justification Sheet: Critical Path
and Integrated Progress Note 77

Figure 3-11. Newton-Wellesley Time Line (in Retrospect) 78

Figure 3-12. Enhanced Delivery System: Key Components 79

Figure 3-13. Patient Processing System 80

Figure 3-14. Care Management and Case Management:
Improvement Measures 83

Figure 3-15. Care Management and Case Management:
Resource Consumption 83

Figure 3-16. The Miriam Hospital Case Management
AMI Patient Outcome Audit Tool: DRG 122 85

Figure 3-17. The Miriam Hospital Patient Satisfaction Report:
Case Management Program 86

Figure 3-18. Clinical Improvement Team/High-Level Flow 87

Figure 3-19. Coordinated Care Program Key Components 89

Figure 3-20. MBMC Coordinated Care Steering Committee 89

Figure 3-21. Coordinated Care Program Evaluation Budget 92

Figure 4-1. Project Management: CareMap Project Phases 96

Figure 4-2. Characteristics of a Fully Integrated CareMap
and/or Case Management System 107

Figure 4-3. Project Management: Sample Time Line 108

Figure 4-4. Project Management: Sample Project Manager
Role Functions 108

Figure 5-1. Descriptive Categories for Case Type Populations 116

Figure 5-2. Roles, Tasks, and Responsibilities That Support
a Productive Mapping Process 117

Figure 5-3. Sample Agenda for CareMap Development Session 118

Figure 5-4. Differentiating Author Team Goals from the
Larger CareMap Program Initiative Goals 121

Figure 5-5. The CareMap Grid and Elements to Complete
in a Development Session 121

Figure   5-6.   CareMap Columns Used to Display Time Progression
                and Location Changes 122

Figure   5-7.   Defining Accountability for Tasks and Outcomes
                within the Grid Cells 123

Figure   5-8.   Common Start-Up Questions and Short Answers
                for a CareMap Tool Pilot 125

Figure   5-9.   Process for Authoring, Ratifying, and Revising
                CareMap Tools 126

Figure 5-10.   JCAHO Emphasis in the Agenda for Change Initiative
                and Correlating Features in CareMap Tools and Systems 128

Figure   6-1.   Bell Curve Distribution Showing Effect
                of Managed Care Model Using CareMap 133

Figure   6-2.   Care Path® for Thoracotomy 137

Figure   6-3.   Care Path® Variance Tracking Form 142

Figure   6-4.   Variance Source Codes 144

Figure   6-5.   Variance Report by Category of Care 145

Figure   6-6.   Positive/Negative Variance Comparison Report 146

Figure   6-7.   CareMap Improvement Opportunities 146

Figure   7-1.   Total Knee CareMap Document (Excerpt) 155

Figure   7-2.   Illustration of Signature Log and Initial Column
                Tied to Date Columns 156

Figure   7-3.   Illustration of Signature Tied to Initialed Date Columns
                on Separate Page from the Map 157

Figure   7-4.   Illustration of Signature Log at Base of Intervention Columns . . . 158

Figure   8-1.   Care over the Continuum 166

Figure   8-2.   Dimensions of and Strategies for Care Coordination 167

Figure   8-3.   Expanding Scope of Accountability 168

Figure   8-4.   Case Management Models 169

Figure   8-5.   Case Manager Role Functions 171

Figure   8-6.   Minimal Knowledge and Skill Components
                of the Case Manager's Role 172

Figure   8-7.   Sample Case Management Network 173

Figure   8-8.   Anatomy of an Effective Case Management Design 176

Figure   9-1.   Case Management as a Bottom-Line Management
                and Quality of Care Delivery Model: Features of the Process
                and Their Relationship with Model Outcomes 178

Figure   9-2.   Tools for Evaluating Program Outcomes 182

Figure 10-1.   Evolution from Current Practice to Automated Ideal Practice . . . 199

Figure 10-2.   Comparison of Case Management Profiles: Utilization Review
                and Clinical Nursing Departments 203

About the Editor

Karen Zander, MS, CS, CS, is a principal in The Center for Case Management at South Natick, Massachusetts. Previously, she held a variety of positions over a period of 19 years with New England Medical Center Hospitals in Boston, including nurse manager, staff education instructor, clinical supervisor, and organizational development specialist. Her pioneering work with case management and CareMap systems is internationally recognized. Ms. Zander has published extensively in periodicals and textbooks, and has been the editor of *The New Definition* for 10 years. She is copublisher, along with Kathleen Bower, of *Issues and Outcomes,* the newsletter for mapping and managing care. Ms. Zander also maintains a private practice in psychotherapy and is certified by the American Nurses' Association.

Contributors

Kathleen M. Andolina, RN, MS, CS, is a consultant for The Center for Case Management at South Natick, Massachusetts, where she works with health care facilities starting collaborative case management programs using CareMap tools and critical paths. She also teaches in a BSN nursing program at the Massachusetts College of Pharmacy and Allied Health Sciences in Boston, and is developing a master's degree program in outcomes-based practice. Additionally, Ms. Andolina is a clinical specialist in psychiatric mental health and frequently speaks on issues related to coordinated care and outcomes practice in mental health.

Kathleen Bower, DNSc, RN, is a principal in The Center for Case Management at South Natick, Massachusetts. Previously, she held a series of positions over a period of 17 years at New England Medical Center Hospitals in Boston. She pioneered the development of nursing case management at NEMC and has since helped organizations in the U.S., Canada, Australia, and England implement and refine critical path/CareMap and case management systems. Recent publications include *Case Management by Nurses* (American Nurses Association, 1992) and chapters in *The Encyclopedia of Nursing Care Quality* (Aspen, 1991) and *The Physician Leader's Guide* (Bader and Associates, 1992).

Judith L. Brett, RN, MSN, PhD, is vice-president, Ancillary Services, at Robert Wood Johnson University Hospital in New Brunswick, New Jersey. Dr. Brett has held a variety of health care service roles in nursing research, management, and education as well as hospital administration. Her areas of expertise include quality of care and outcomes measurement and management, work redesign for nursing and hospital organizations, and nursing systems evaluation and design.

Maria Hill, RN, MSN, is a senior consultant at The Center for Case Management at South Natick, Massachusetts. Previously, she held various positions over a period of 10 years at University Hospital and Clinics in Madison, Wisconsin. Her experience includes all aspects of program design, implementation, maintenance, and evaluation. Contributions to several books include CareMap and Case Management Systems: Evolving Models Designed to Enhance Patient Care, in: *Redesigning Nursing Care Delivery: Transforming Our Future* (J. B. Lippincott, 1994); Integrating Critical Pathways and

Documentation by Exception, in: *Charting by Exception Applications* (Delmar Publishers, 1995); and Integration of Managed Care with Informational Systems, in: *Information Management: Strategies and Support for Data Driven Decisions in Nursing and Health Care* (Springhouse Corporation, 1995).

John Kleinman, MD, FACP, is group vice-president, professional services group, Allina Health System, Minneapolis. From 1988 until 1994 he was vice-president for medical affairs, Mercy and Unity Hospitals, HealthSpan Health System Corporation. Dr. Kleinman has been a member of the clinical faculty of the University of Minnesota's Departments of Medicine and Family Practice and currently is a Fellow of the American College of Physicians. He is also a member of the Minnesota Medical Association, the Hennepin County Medical Society, and the American College of Physician Executives. From 1985 through 1994 Dr. Kleinman was a member of Blue Plus, Blue Cross/Blue Shield of Minnesota's Board of Directors' Formulary Committee and was chair of their Metropolitan Health Care Organization Advisory Council. He also is chair of the Quality Management/Quality Assurance Committee for SelectCare, a Minnesota preferred provider organization.

Susan P. Kyzer, MS, RN, is a senior consultant at The Center for Case Management at South Natick, Massachusetts (based in Greenville, South Carolina). Most recently, she has served as case management project director of a 60-bed pediatric orthopedic hospital, where she is responsible for the development, implementation, and integration of case management and has achieved the goal of having all patient care managed via the CareMap system. Ms. Kyzer has dealt extensively with issues involving the integration of CareMap systems with documentation, variance analysis, and quality improvement.

Patricia Potter, RN, MSN, is director of nursing practice at Barnes and Jewish Hospitals in St. Louis, Missouri. She has directed the hospital's care path program for the past four years as well as lead in the development and evaluation of delivery of care models, nursing standards of practice, and quality improvement initiatives. Ms. Potter serves as a part-time consultant for The Center for Case Management in South Natick, Massachusetts, and is coauthor of numerous nursing fundamentals textbooks.

Mary Crabtree Tonges, RN, MSN, MBA, is a consultant with The Center for Case Management, in South Natick, Massachusetts. She is an author and speaker on nursing administration, with particular expertise in work redesign and alternative nursing practice and care delivery models. She has held nurse executive positions at Robert Wood Johnson University Hospital in New Brunswick, New Jersey, and Northwestern Memorial Hospital in Chicago. Ms. Tonges is a Commonwealth Fund Executive Nurse Fellow and currently is a doctoral student in organization and policy studies at Baruch College of the City University of New York.

Preface

I have always been skeptical of new systems that are process heavy and are not linked to tangible, positive results for patients and their families. Unlike other change strategies, CareMap® tools and provider-controlled case management models have been developed to directly structure the management of outcomes by formalizing positive, collaborative processes. These strategies have stood the test of time as well as the test of multiple applications by clinicians around the world. In most cases, CareMap tools and case management models have provided hope, control, and a newfound synergy among professional disciplines, departments, and agencies. CareMap tools and case management models will carry health care organizations into the next century as health care adapts to or aggressively embraces the continuum of care and capitation arrangements. CareMap tools and case management models are offered in this text as a bridge to the art, science, and business of health care.

This book reflects the way CareMap and case management projects have evolved in health care organizations. Chapter 1 brings the reader up-to-date with a description of these strategies, which are grounded in principles of good care and its efficient, collaborative management. An historical perspective of critical paths and case management leads logically to their contemporary relationship with major trends in health care. Chapter 2 emphasizes the current health care agenda from the physician's perspective and discusses the practical need for physician leadership as well as its academic foundation.

Chapter 3 addresses the need for precise project planning, and ultimately program design, that reflects an organization's mission. Making "models" realistic, having an executive steering committee, and using collaborative, self-managed teams at several levels is described in theory and in practice.

Chapters 4 and 5 describe the detailed work of project management and collaborative CareMap tool development. Strategies for avoiding or overcoming common pitfalls are offered in each chapter.

The documentation of variance (or exception) is the most misunderstood component of collaborative care programs. Both the concurrent clinical use and the retrospective uses of variance are explained in depth in chapter 6. Chapter 7 describes principles by which organizations can begin to integrate the CareMap tool as the core of the

---

CareMap® is a registered trademark of The Center for Case Management, South Natick, MA.

medical record. Characteristics of a fully automated medical record system as well as actual advances in patient education using a CareMap methodology are also offered.

Chapter 8 explores the custom design of a case management model across a continuum of care, spanning health–illness, time, and location. This chapter presents ideas for integrating the best features of diverse applications that now exist.

Chapter 9 on program evaluation suggests that organizations "begin at the end," in other words, establish expected criteria to measure the degree of success of collaborative care while the project is in the formative stages. Frameworks to design, implement, and revise a CareMap and/or case management program evaluation are explained. Actual qualitative and quantitative data from health care literature are discussed as well.

Chapter 10 begins with health care as we know it today and takes it the next logical step by using CareMaps and case management as the bridge. Clinicians' collaboration at many levels is as important as clinicians' skills at achieving desired outcomes for patients and their families. The two pieces of unfinished business in our current endeavors are the need for automation and revised structures for assisting and ensuring accountability.

Acknowledgments

Karen Zander and Kathleen Bower, principals of The Center for Case Management, would like to thank the staff of American Hospital Publishing, Inc., especially Audrey Kaufman, for providing this opportunity to present our collective work spanning the past 10 years. We would not have been able to do this without the goodwill, courage, and advice we receive from our clients, who are implementing CareMap and case management strategies. A special thanks goes to those people and organizations credited in the text who contributed their stories, examples, and recommendations.

The entire staff of The Center for Case Management was involved in writing this text, and we are grateful to them and proud to present their knowledge to you. We are also, as always, indebted to the diligent administrative and moral support of Robyn Ripley, executive administrator, and Dana Corrente, client services coordinator. We are hopeful that our collaborative efforts have produced an outcome that will be helpful to each reader.

CHAPTER ONE

Collaborative Care: Two Effective Strategies for Positive Outcomes

Karen Zander

Since its emergence in health care in 1985, collaborative care has come of age. It is operationalized by two central methodologies: (1) critical paths or their second generation, CareMap® systems; and (2) case management. These specific methodologies represent an acknowledgment of the industry's need for clinical systems that manage patient care toward positive, measurable outcomes within a cost-effective framework. Critical paths/CareMap tools and case management create an infrastructure that can be implemented and evaluated on many levels. Because they can produce far-reaching changes in, first, the process and, second, the structure of care provision, they should be understood conceptually and historically.

This chapter provides a definition for collaborative care and describes the two principal strategies that operationalize it: critical paths/CareMap systems and case management. It also describes the historical development of these strategies, principally as practiced by the nursing staff at New England Medical Center Hospitals in Boston, and explains the relationship between these collaborative care strategies and trends in health care.

Collaborative Care

The concept of collaborative care is not new. However, with the recognition that individual professionals and departments are highly interdependent has finally come the realization that achievement of financial efficiency and clinical effectiveness also is a matter of interdependency. Growing numbers of health care providers now recognize that collaboration helps focus interdependent processes on priorities and practical solutions that move patients toward their optimal outcomes.

People collaborate when they perceive, or are held to, a mutual purpose or goal. In this text, *collaborative care* is defined as "inclusionary care," in which all care providers and receivers of care are involved at the highest level possible. In collaborative care, all players are given maximum authority to define and carry out their responsibilities. Through authority there is accountability; therefore, collaborative care is accountable care. In other words, rather than being an end in itself, collaborative care

CareMap® is a registered trademark of The Center for Case Management, South Natick, MA.

is a *condition* of an accountable practice in which desired patient/family outcomes are the uniting force. As such, it is the practice of mature clinicians of every profession. Indeed, much of patient care requires working with at least one other professional if not scores of information and support staff to achieve the patient goals for which the clinician is accountable.

Formal methods for collaborative practice, especially between nurses and physicians, have been studied periodically. The largest study was done between 1971 and 1981 by the National Joint Practice Commission (NJPC), an interprofessional organization to improve health care established by action of the American Medical Association and the American Nurses' Association.[1] The study identified five elements that were key to joint or collaborative practice:

1. A joint practice committee
2. Primary nursing
3. Individual nurse clinical decision making
4. Integrated patient care records
5. Joint patient care record review

Although the NJPC gave sound advice, few institutions implemented its findings either in part or at all, probably due to a lack of financial or political pressure from external sources. In retrospect, institutions may have perceived that collaborative practice would require more time and resources internally. Additionally, collaborative practice as an end in itself obviously was not a goal of all parties. To this day, collaboration (if present) generally is considered a bonus to practice rather than a fair expectation of practice. Each discipline wants cooperation and support, but often anticipates and experiences conflict in its relationships with others. In fact, many would say that the health care team concept is more myth than reality. Clinicians feel isolated and sometimes even thwarted in their attempts to respond to patient needs. Without relatively straightforward mechanisms to develop and maintain it, collaboration quickly disappears under the stress of the work environment.

Critical paths/CareMap systems and case management have provided the necessary mechanisms to make collaborative care a reality. The current need to control costs and discover reliable quality processes is forcing health care agencies to find the time for collaborative planning and restructuring. Perhaps there is a subtle but definite difference between *collaborative practice* — as a mechanism of professionals' relationships with each other — and *collaborative care* — as a mechanism for achieving patients' and families' outcomes in an era when collaboration promotes survival rather than mere luxury. Indeed, it is the intense mandate to focus on outcomes that will drive the acceptance and adoption of collaborative care methods in every care setting.

Precursors to Collaborative Care

The history of critical path/CareMap tools and case management strategies depends on who is asked! As with all classic models, collaborative care has roots in sound theory and practice and represents a convergence and reintegration of separate ideas. At the risk of oversimplifying history, it could be said that critical paths grew out of industrial engineering and project management and that case management emerged from public health and social welfare approaches for procuring basic resources (fuel, shelter, food) for people in need.

A more detailed, but by no means extensive, time line appears in figure 1-1, representing estimates in trends that have contributed to or influenced the evolution of collaborative care practice. As the time line shows, access to care as well as regulation of caregiver credentials and eventually of organizations is a constant theme beginning in the first half of this century. Formal methods for the payment of care by

Figure 1-1. Evolution of Trends toward Collaborative Care

Late 1800s	Social welfare and conscience
1900	"Cases" of MDs, lawyers, public health nurses
1910	
1920	State licensure laws, peer review
1930	JCAHO founded
1940	Clinical case audit
1945	Psychiatric nurses "case-manage" WW II veterans
1950	Workers' Compensation, community mental health centers, space industry critical paths, matrix management
1960	
1965	Medicare–Medicaid became law First-generation severity measurement systems
1970	Primary nursing
1972	Professional Standards Review Organizations, Utilization Law Review
1975	JCAHO retrospective outcome audit criteria Insurance company case managers
1980	HMOs
1981	
1983	DRGs
1985	Case management plans, NEMCH
1986	Acute care case managers, NEMCH Critical paths, NEMCH
1989	CareMap systems first implemented RWJ/PEW grants to strengthen hospital nursing Agency for Healthcare Policy and Research established, with Medical Treatment Initiatives Program
1990	CQI, TQM
1991	
1992	
1993	AHA Quality Measurement and Management Project 15,000 certified case managers in U.S. JCAHO Agenda for Change
1994	

Sources:

Development of Case Management Models. Systemedics: Little Rock, Arkansas (Handout).

Halfar, A. Healthcare quality measurement technology development. *The New Definition* 7(2):1, Spring 1992.

Nash, D. The state of the outcomes/guidelines movement. *Decisions in Imaging Economics* 6(2)11–20, Spring 1993.

insurers, the government, health maintenance organizations (HMOs), and so on became more influential trends in the second half of the century. It is interesting to note that there were few changes in the way institutional patient care was organized and managed until the advent of primary nursing in the late 1960s and case management in the mid-1980s.

The medical model, in which the physician's orders are assumed to account for and guide all patient care needs from diagnosis and treatment through recovery and recuperation, remains predominant throughout the century. Although this may be a faulty assumption, it is at the core of most strategies for health care policy and reform. CareMap tools and case management, combined with continuous quality improvement (CQI), although encompassing the medical model, provide a more comprehensive set of processes and solutions to improve systems of health care delivery than does the medical model or regulation alone. In other words, collaboration at the care-giving level probably will have more impact on caregivers than regulations, payers, and other external influences will have.

The Pratt 4 Project

One precursor to the development of collaborative care via critical paths/CareMap tools and case management at New England Medical Center Hospitals (NEMCH) in Boston was the Pratt 4 Project, conducted in 1983. It was undertaken to study how the care provided by Pratt 4, a surgical unit, could be improved while using the same or decreased resources. A socio-technical-environmental analysis technique was used by a multidisciplinary study team.[2]

As in subsequent process analyses in many organizations since that time, areas of ambiguity and inefficiencies were identified. Just as important, certain unexpected "truths" emerged in 1983 about care giving in and beyond acute care. Listed below, they greatly contributed to the direction and manner in which collaborative care was formulated two years later.

- *Describing the work of a hospital by geographic unit was only a partial view of reality.* For example, whereas nursing was organized by unit, the physicians' primary allegiance was to their practice or service and all other professionals had primary allegiance to their departments. Thus, the only common denominator between these diverse players was that of groupings of homogeneous populations, or *case types.* (See figure 1-2.)
- *Physicians usually were not willing to represent other physicians at meetings or committees.* They also had low tolerance for "process-heavy" meetings—that is, meetings lacking a clear task and outcome.
- *Clinicians came to work expecting to "do battle" with each other and with unresponsive support services.* Flow diagrams of processes revealed many slowdowns and frustrations in the delivery of multiservices from admission to discharge.
- *The foundation of the way care per patient was organized needed change.* This was true even if more staff were added to the unit or if tasks were shifted to other departments. Without more useful tools for care management and more reliable working relationships between the clinical decision makers, all other changes would be little more than window dressing.
- *Defining the cost of care only in terms of resources ordered by a physician was an inadequate formula.* Nurses and others had a major role in detecting patient needs and asking physicians to render decisions and orders.

Perhaps the most important lesson of the Pratt 4 Project was that clinicians saw themselves as working for the patient and family, even though each discipline and

Figure 1-2. Case Type as Common Denominator

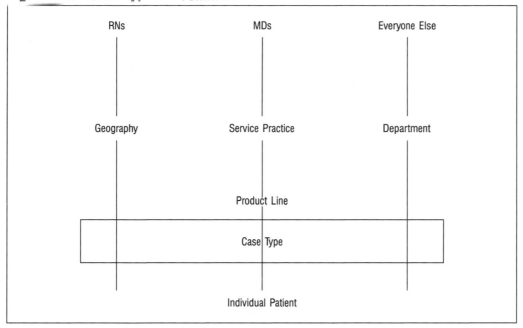

department interpreted the content and goals of the work differently and was more or less removed from a position of authority to act on information. Everyone felt responsible for doing a good job and had learned how to work around policies and edicts that were not facilitative of immediate patient goals. It was clear that any new major clinical program could not be imposed on the current situation and that any new program would have to be built from the clinical work outward for managers and administrators to support it.

By 1985, it was clear that the restructuring of the relationship between time, money, and manpower in health care, best characterized by the onset of diagnosis-related groups (DRGs), created NEMCH's best and possibly last opportunity to define, price, evaluate, and develop professional clinician contribution. Leadership in practice would entail the articulation, management, and research of the clinical outcomes resulting from sound assessments, diagnoses, plans, and processes. This mission would be complex, especially because clinical outcomes can occur randomly, unpredictably, and out of context to the patients' and families' real concerns. Yet, future evaluation and research of practice would be almost impossible unless outcomes were structured into the fabric of each professional's role.

Critical Paths and Their Next Generation

Collaborative care via critical paths and case management was introduced into acute care by the nurses at NEMCH in 1985. This application emerged from the concern that, due to DRGs, acute care agencies would lose control and autonomy over what they knew was good practice. Without a structure and response to the push to decrease length of stay (LOS) and resources, patient and family outcomes might be jeopardized.

Nurses were the most likely candidates to introduce critical paths and case management because they are at the juncture where the system and the patient meet. Nurses have to either make the larger system work for the patient or directly experience the patient's anger, pain, and complications related to inefficient or ineffective activities. Also, through the applied scientific method they call the *nursing process,* nurses use nomenclature that breaks the medical diagnosis into workable, treatable parts (that is, into the nursing diagnosis), which in turn can make a conceptual bridge to outcome definition. In addition, accountability models such as primary nursing give nurses a background to begin a collaborative dialogue. Thus, with a sound structure in place, the nurses at NEMCH had the confidence to ask the following four questions of all disciplines:

1. What is the work required to get patients within certain case types to desired outcomes?
2. What is the best way to produce the work, including clinical decision making (academic, crisis, structured process) and a model/structure (people for care giving, responsibilities, relationships, documentation)?
3. Who is accountable for the results?
4. What do we need to restructure to better support our clinical processes?

To begin, the conceptual link was made between cost, process, and outcome. Each had to be in balance with the other; neither could be investigated out of context of the other two components.

Between 1985 and 1989, four designs of written documents for planning, managing, documenting, and evaluating multidisciplinary care toward outcomes evolved as more was learned about outcome-based clinical care within time frames. Each iteration of design created more confidence in the need and ability to move from open-ended care planning to structured care managing. Along with the documents went experimentation with case management roles and structures.

Design #1. Case Management Plans

Case management plans (CMPs) were the first attempt to capture patterns of care processes and then define outcomes that would be written against a time standard and used to manage care. They included four broad categories of clinical outcome ("products" in an industrial engineering model), with three related outcomes of cost, LOS, and patient/family satisfaction. The four outcome categories used were from the Joint Commission on Accreditation of Healthcare Organizations's (JCAHO's) retrospective audit criteria: health, knowledge, activity/function, and absence of complications.

- *Health outcomes:* Optimal and realistic physical or emotional conditions of patients that could be anticipated at discharge or transfer from a care area. These outcomes should be at least partially influenced by interventions.
- *Knowledge outcomes:* Stated as the completion of appropriate formal teaching plans and/or the demonstration of specific learning goals not on available teaching plans.
- *Activity (physical/role function) outcomes:* Attainable behaviors of the patient/family that indicate adaptation to the change or a return to normal baseline functioning.
- *Absence of complication outcomes:* Absence of potential problems found on assessment and/or known to be common for the case type.

Overall, the CMPs described the following elements for each DRG (or its derivative) within a major diagnostic category:

- Problem/focus/nursing diagnoses and their related outcomes within each broad outcome category. These are the usual, expected diagnoses and outcomes encountered by 90 percent of patients/families within the specific DRG.
- Intermediate goals and the processes (interventions, tasks) needed to achieve them.

- Time frames in intervals of hours, days, weeks, or numbers of visits within which processes must occur to meet anticipated intermediate goals.

It was planned that with computerization, each CMP would have maximum capability of individualizing any of the above elements based on initial and ongoing assessments. However, computerization of these extensive plans was deemed impossible at the time, so paper CMPs were trialed.

Thirty-five CMPs were developed at NEMCH using a standard methodology. To design them, clinical managers investigated variables affecting LOS, cause-and-effect relationships between tasks and outcomes, and concurrent audits to assess the degree to which clinicians managed patients and their families toward predetermined outcomes.

An excerpt from a CMP for a patient diagnosed with idiopathic pediatric scoliosis is shown in figure 1-3. As the figure shows, the CMP outlines the relationship between time, manpower, and cost as they converge to produce measurable outcomes, which are actually behaviorally measured standards. As opposed to open-ended care plans, CMPs were a tool to control interventions and their subsequent outcomes on a time-prescribed basis. Interventions were outlined so specifically that they could be associated with patient classification measures of acuity and cost. Thus, hypothetically, the CMP achieved many goals for health care, including:

- Development of clinical product lines with related costs per outcome rather than per task, which enabled resources to be understood in a new, more defined and professional context
- Daily control over outcomes and their interventions, both measurable yet able to be revised
- Establishment of potential contracts among nurses, patients, families, physicians, and health care institutions
- Integration of planning, managing, documenting, and pricing
- Development of a common base for research among caregivers, units, and institutions (currently called *benchmarking*)

Physician process data were first piloted with the scoliosis CMP. This case type was selected because of an existing (though informal) protocol for these patients. Also, the nursing staff on the pediatric surgical unit had already developed a successful collaborative relationship with the attending staff. Because of the success of this pilot, the authors of other CMPs were asked to work with an attending physician from the appropriate service to develop the physician component for their case type. A variety of responses and issues emerged from the nurses and physicians involved.

From the nursing perspective, some of the factors considered when identifying the physician to participate included:

- How the request might be perceived in light of pressures and changes occurring inside the institution or outside
- Which physician(s) usually cared for patients of that case type
- The strength of the collaborative relationship between that physician group and the nursing staff
- The degree to which physician practices vary with the population
- Who had authority to develop a standard protocol in the event that practices do vary greatly
- Whether the person with the authority has an interest or investment in developing a standard protocol

Although some physicians were reluctant to participate in content development (interpreting the move as a possible precursor to yet another control of their practice),

Figure 1-3. Case Management Plan Excerpt: Scoliosis

DIAGNOSIS: Idiopathic Pediatric Scoliosis, with surgery, without complications   UNIT: **Floating 7 South**   DRG: **215**

MDC: **8**   LENGTH OF STAY: **14 days**   USUAL OR DAY (from admission day = 1): **3**

HEALTH OUTCOMES

DIAGNOSIS	OUTCOME (The patient . . .)	DAY VISIT	INTERMEDIATE GOAL (The patient . . .)	DAY VISIT	PROCESS (The nurse . . .)	DAY VISIT	PROCESS (The physician . . .)	DAY VISIT
Fluid/electrolyte imbalance; third space shifting secondary to large volume loss and replacement	• Vital signs are stable and consistent with admission baseline.	5–6	• Is afebrile. • Maintains VS within the following range: P ___ BP ___ R ___ T ___	5–6 4–14	• Takes vital signs q2h for 8h post op then q4h if patient afebrile and vital signs stable, then q shift. • Notifies MD if P > ___, BP > ___, R > ___, T > ___, or if P < ___, BP < ___, R < ___, T < ___.	4 5–9 10–14 1–14	• Upon family's request arranges for self blood donation by patient over a 3–4 month period.	PTA
							• On admission assesses the patient's cardiac status. Orders an EKG. Reviews cardiac landmarks on Scoli series. If there is evidence or history of abnormality or compromise an echocardiogram and/or cardiology consult may be ordered.	1
	• Voiding pattern is at baseline normal.		• Maintains urine output over 1cc/KG/hr while Foley catheter in. • Voids 8 hours after Foley is discontinued. • Maintains Specific Gravity under .1020.	4–6 6–7 4–14	• Measures and records I/O q1h for 24h, then q4h if stable (while Foley in), then every shift. • Notifies MD if output under ___ cc/hr while Foley in. • Monitors specific gravity q2h for 8h, q4h for 48h if stable, then every shift. • Notifies MD if SG over .1020. • Calculates 24h I/O for OR day on return to unit.	4 5–6 7–14 4–6 5–6 7–14 4–14 4	• Orders the following lab studies CBC with differential PT, PTT, Platelet Count, BUN, Creatinine, Urinalysis with Sediment.	1
	• Has no edema.		• Returns to baseline skin turgor.	8–9	• Balances IV and oral intake to achieve maintenance fluid requirements, then forces oral fluids to maintenance. • Observes dressing when patient turned and notifies MD of new or increased bloody staining. • Empties and records hemovac drainage q4-8h. Notifies MD of drainage over 100cc in 4h.	4–8 9–14 4–10 4–7	• Orders a bleeding time if there is a suggestive history and/or abnormal coagulation studies. • Types and crossmatches the patient for appropriate volume of blood based on weight and exact procedure to be done (usually 6-8 units in adolescent patients).	PRN 24th Prior to OR

Reprinted, with permission, from Stetler, C., and DeZell, A. D. Case Management Plans: Designs for Transformation. Boston: New England Medical Center Hospitals, 1987, pp. 26–32.

others were already practicing by protocol and saw their participation as an opportunity to ensure continuity. Still others saw it as a means of influencing changes to come. Most were quick to see the value of the CMPs as teaching tools for new multidisciplinary staff.

Once committed, physicians voiced some common concerns. They needed some of the same educational support that nurses had needed in understanding how to clearly define and differentiate patient problems and the corresponding intermediate goals and outcomes. They also anticipated some difficulty in designating specific time frames, though they could list the usual treatment regime and the necessary sequence of events for a particular case type. Most physicians had limited knowledge of Health Care Financing Administration (HCFA) LOS statistics and some were surprised at the historic LOS data for NEMCH, obtained from the finance database. They expressed the need to account for the variables that affected practice.

NEMCH attributed initial success to the straightforward presentation of its goal: to establish a patient-centered care delivery system that would achieve cost-effective care within established standards. This appealed to the physicians' own concerns about quality and offered a concrete tool for monitoring and controlling quality while still responding to the mounting pressure to decrease LOS and resource utilization.

All these changes required tremendous coordination and teaching efforts as well as ongoing communication and contact between professionals and with patients. Physicians acknowledged that nurses were vital in this environment. Additionally, physicians were acutely aware that they must become more competitive and progressive in their approach to care as preferred provider organizations (PPOs) and discount pricing structures continued to evolve. The CMP model offered new marketing potential in these arenas.[3]

Design #2. Time Lines

Although CMPs were very helpful for guiding the collaborative interventions for a patient on one unit, because of the specialization of nursing units, they did not address the tasks or outcomes for patients who needed care on several units during their hospital stay. Time lines were the documents that helped NEMCH make the transition from unit-based care to case-based care management. In their most basic form, time lines were one-line diagrams identifying predictable clinical landmarks and the associated time intervals for an episode of illness. For example, the typical perinatal time line comprises 9 months for prenatal visits, 4 to 24 hours for labor and delivery, 2 days for postpartum care, and time for one or more follow-up visits.[4]

In their more detailed form, time lines show the key patient problems for a specific case type or DRG. In addition, they include related, expected outcomes in each of the categories discussed earlier to be accomplished in each geographic unit.

The standard outcomes included in the time lines were set and met in collaboration with physicians, patients/families, and other health care professionals. An excerpt of the time line for uncomplicated myocardial infarction (DRG 122) is shown in figure 1-4. In addition to the intermediate goals for each outcome in each geographic unit, the most detailed time line describes the processes (interventions) within the time intervals to be accomplished by nurses, physicians, and others. Both processes and goals are displayed serially to reflect the patient's transfer from unit to unit.

Although time lines were not new to health care, their formalization per case type as a protocol for every associated care unit was long overdue. With few exceptions, not too long ago the bed to which a patient was admitted was the bed from which he or she was discharged. With the onset of intensive care units (ICUs) and subspecialties, patient transfers from one care area to another has become the everyday reality. The mental and monetary expense of fragmented acute care is ever present.

Continuity of care was always a challenge not only within one unit during 24 hours, but also between multiple units within one hospital. Although the physician

Figure 1-4. Excerpts from Time Line Overview: Uncomplicated MI (DRG 122)

Emergency Room Day 1	Coronary Care Unit 2 3	Inpatient Cardiology 4 5 6 7 8 9 10	Outpatient Cardiology Visit 1 2
Health Outcomes			
1. DX: Alteration in comfort secondary to chest pain.	1. DX: Alteration in comfort secondary to chest pain.	1. DX: Alteration in comfort secondary to chest pain.	1. DX: Potential alteration in comfort secondary to chest pain.
Outcome: Chest pain is controlled by IV nitroglycerin, nitrates, oxygen, and/or morphine. Rates each episode of chest pain using a 1–10 severity scale.	Outcome: Is free of chest pain or pain is controlled by three or fewer sublingual nitroglycerin tablets. Rates each episode of chest pain on a 1–10 severity scale.	Outcome: Chest pain is controlled by three or fewer sublingual nitroglycerin tablets.	Outcome: Controls pain with prophylactic medication management, and reports changes in frequency and nature of chest pain to care provider.
Nurse-Dependent Complications			
1. DX: Potential for untoward effects of medications.	1. DX: Potential for untoward effects of medications.	1. DX: Potential for untoward effects of medications.	1. DX: Potential for untoward effects of an alteration in cardiac status secondary to medication regimen.
Outcome: Demonstrates no untoward effects of medications, including mental status changes, tachycardia, or hypotension.	Outcome: Demonstrates no untoward effects of medications, including mental status changes, hypotension, tachycardia, or bleeding.	Outcome: Demonstrates no adverse side effects including mental status changes, hypotension, tachycardia, or bleeding.	Outcome: Takes medications as scheduled as measured by response to medications and patient self-report. Reports medication intolerance to care provider.
Activity Outcomes			
1. DX: Restrictions in activity secondary to rule out MI.	1. DX: Restrictions in activity secondary to MI.	1. DX: Restrictions in ADLs secondary to MI.	1. DX: Alterations in ADLs secondary to MI.
Outcome: Maintains bed rest.	Outcome: Tolerates sitting in chair, bathing, feeding self, reading, watching TV without chest pain, shortness of breath, or tachycardia.	Outcome: Ambulates ad lib and completes activities of daily living without chest pain or chest pain that is controlled by nitroglycerin.	Outcome: Modifies former lifestyle to control chest pain or chest pain is controlled by p.o. nitroglycerin.
Knowledge Outcomes			
1. DX: Knowledge deficit related to hospitalization and chest pain.	1. DX: Knowledge deficit related to ICU hospitalization and MI.	1. DX: Knowledge deficit related to MI and posthospital self-care.	1. DX: Knowledge deficit related to coronary artery disease.
Outcome: States is being admitted to the hospital and gives a simple reason for hospitalization.	Outcome: Meets the objectives of the following teaching plans: orientation to CCU, primary nursing, and sections of the congestive heart failure, MI, and angina teaching plans.	Outcome: Meets the objectives of the MI and angina teaching plans.	Outcome: Upon review, meets the objectives of the MI and angina teaching plans.
			2. DX: Knowledge deficit related to controllable risk factors.
			Outcome: Identifies own risk factors. Institutes activities to control risk factors.

Source: Bower, K. Case management: meeting the challenge. *Definition* 3(1):3, Winter 1988. Used with permission.

and medical record usually travel with the patient, there is minimal opportunity in terms of time or institutional sanction to prescribe nursing processes or interventions across a continuum of care. Because nurses are geographically based, even primary nurses cannot have the entire perspective, control, or feedback regarding course of treatment. Nurses could not confidently tell a patient or family what lay ahead. Subsequently, nurses felt isolated as well as pressured to complete every function (such as patient teaching) during their time with the patient. Thus, patient care was at risk of omission or duplication as the number of transfers multiplied. In whatever level of detail, time lines cannot help but increase everyone's sense of security and control.

Time lines for over 20 major case types or DRGs were developed at NEMCH. All were completed in collaboration with two or more geographic patient care units, using current nurse and physician practice patterns as the reference point. In many cases, the same patient problems held true across all clinical areas. This occurred even though outcomes and related processes might have differed.

The purpose of this first set of time lines was not to create a perfect scenario with perfect wording but, rather, to capture and chart current practice and the language used to describe it. The insights and respect gained between clinicians and managers in geographically separated areas was as important as the documents they produced.

Time lines provided clinicians, managers, administrators, and, ultimately, patients and their families with a clearer definition of health care. They raised new, exciting, and challenging questions, including:

- How far does accountability for outcomes extend, because nursing and other services tend to be unit based whereas cost-per-case strategies must transcend an individual unit?
- Can time lines assist in the accurate estimation of nursing and other budgets, new patient care programs (product line management), or better timing of processes (interventions)?
- To what degree should patients be made aware of their predicted time lines?
- How can time lines stimulate meaningful research?
- What kind of management support do future case managers need?

Time lines were a valuable step in the response to the advent of managed care. They added new meaning to the goal of continuity of care and the necessity to expand and empower roles, and both rattled caregiver needs for "turf." Although they could never replace the skill, judgment, or compassion of clinicians, time lines helped chart the way for true patient-centered care.

Design #3. Critical Paths

Ironically, critical paths were a fallback strategy because CMPs and time lines were too unwieldy to use clinically and because computerization was still a long way off. Therefore, critical paths were minimalist reminder sheets for clinicians in tracking and coordinating resources with the assumption that intermediate and discharge outcomes would occur if interventions were applied appropriately.

A *critical path* is a standardized, prewritten, one- or two-page document showing the interventions of all disciplines along a time schedule. (See figure 1-5.) In effect, it is a grid, with time as one axis and staff actions as the other.

Because critical paths were nonconceptual, visually appealing, relatively easy to write, and effective in reviewing and often decreasing LOS, they gained international attention quickly. They were applied to a wide variety of situations, often starting with orthopedic and open-heart surgical procedures and then expanding to less-predictable case types such as asthma, a subset (for example, asthma in children in the emergency department), or a condition (for example, failure to wean).

Figure 1-5. Critical Path and Variance Record: Myocardial Infarction

Patient_____

MD_____

Case Manager_____

Date Critical Path_____

   Reviewed by MD_____

      Date

Case Type Myocardial_____

           Infarction_____

DRG_____122_____

Expected LOS   7 Days

MYOCARDIAL INFARCTION
CRITICAL PATHWAY

	Day 1	Day 2	Day 3	Day 4	Day 5	Day 6	Day 7
ICU	————————————————————— 6S —————————————————————————						
Consults		Cardiac Rehab. Dietician				Copy of Low Chol. No Added Salt Diet	
Tests	EKG	EKG; ETT if nec. for Day 6 Echo, Muga, if nec.	EKG; Receive MBs; R/I or R/O MI; Holter if nec. on Day 5		Holter ETT Cath. if nec.		
Activity	BRP w/ Commode		OOB Chair		Amb in Rm/Hall w/Asst	Up Ad——→ Lib Stairs	
Treatments	O₂ ——————————————————— > D/C O₂						
	Cardiac Monitor ————————————————————————————→					D/C Monitor p negative Holter	
	I & O qd ————————————————————————————→					D/C I & O qd wt, unless CHF	
Medications	IV ——————————— Heparin ————————————————————— > D/C Heparin						
		Lock					Lock
Diet	No Added Salt, Low Chol. Diet ———————————————————————————————→						
Discharge Planning		VNA			Check w/ Attending RE:D/C Date	Discharge Orders	Discharge before 12 Noon
Teaching	Angina, MI, PN., Med, Teaching Plan in Chart	Begin MI Teaching Plan	3 discharge classes Formal Med tx				Amb Classes Re:Risk Factors Diet & smoking

Admission Date_____   Discharge Date_____   Discharge Time_____

   Days in ICU_____   Stress test date_____   Cardiac cath. date_____

   Days in Routine bed_____   Thalium_____

                   Routine_____

            Holter date_____

DATE	VARIATION	CAUSE	ACTION TAKEN

(Reverse side of Critical Pathway form shown above)

Each patient population has a historical LOS and traditional clinical approaches per physician and per institution. These clinical approaches are considered practice patterns, which in turn are rooted in tradition, science, convenience, research, preference, and ethics. Once these practice patterns are discussed among principal players, it is possible to put language to key interventions. In turn, interventions can be classified and written in categories acceptable to the authors. As seen in figure 1-5, critical path categories generally include:

- Consults and assessments
- Tests and specimens
- Activity
- Treatments
- Medications
- Diet
- Discharge coordination
- Teaching

Following is a description of the original authoring and use of critical paths.[5] Although the recommended process of writing and using paths has changed, it is important to understand the initial technique.

Within the first 24 hours of admission to the hospital, a critical path was individualized by the primary nurse and physician, considering comorbidities and psychosocial factors. If changes from the standard were to be made, they were identified at that time. From that point on, all deviations from the critical path were considered *variances*. These were identified on a daily basis and put into three categories of causality—something within the patient, the system, or the caregivers. Any variance was justified by either the primary nurse or attending physician, or action was taken immediately to rectify it.

Critical paths were reviewed by the nursing staff during the change of shift report, three times a day. A report included expected LOS, critical incidents that should occur that day, and variances from the standard. If variances occurred, a primary nurse consultation among the primary nurse's peers was conducted immediately after the report. The critical paths were also used on attending and house officer rounds.

Initially, critical paths were developed to be used directly with patients. Since their development, several equally important ways to utilize them have been discovered—for example, in the orientation of nurses and house staff.

Critical paths were found to be extremely useful in helping clinicians identify targets of opportunity to alter the usual treatment plan for a given case type. They helped to visualize current practice and indicated when either nothing or too much was being done for the patient.

For example, in developing a critical path for patients undergoing induction therapy for leukemia, it was discovered that the usual practice was to admit the patient two to four days before putting in a Cook's catheter. Chemotherapy was then started, followed by antibiotic therapy and/or antifungal therapy for three to four weeks. A complete fever workup was done at least once a day. Electrolytes and blood counts also were drawn daily. A review of subsequent readmissions revealed that the patient was hospitalized four more times for consolidation treatment with chemotherapy.

After examining current practice, the following changes were made:

1. The Cook's catheter was placed on the second day of hospitalization.
2. When the patient was no longer neutropenic and was afebrile, antibiotic therapy and antifungal therapy were completed at home.
3. Mouth care for thrush was begun on the first day, before symptoms become evident.

4. If no new organism was identified, a fever workup was done every 48 hours.
5. Only essential electrolytes and blood counts were drawn on a daily basis.

These changes reduced patient LOS from six to eight weeks (42 to 56 days) to approximately 32 days. The number of unnecessary diagnostic tests also was reduced. In addition, low-dose consolidation chemotherapy is now being given at home, eliminating 14 additional days of hospitalization. Implementation of these changes not only maintained quality outcomes but also improved them. In addition to infection rates being decreased with home chemotherapy, patients slept through the night when a complete fever workup was not done, spent more time with families, and reported increased satisfaction with care and a feeling that they were in better control of what happened to them.

In using critical pathways at NEMCH, it was discovered that:

- Surgical case types are much more likely to follow a standard critical path than are medical case types.
- Medical case types often have other problems during hospitalization that necessitate superimposed critical paths—for example, the patient may have unstable angina and/or angioplasty.
- Adjustment of the standard must always be considered to include comorbidities and psychosocial issues.

NEMCH nurse managers wrote a formal analysis of the relationship between cost, process, and outcome in 1985, and audited the results of the critical path method in 1986. Historically, success of critical paths was measured in one of three ways:[6]

1. Decrease LOS, keeping the same quality outcomes
2. Decrease LOS, increasing the same outcomes
3. Maintain the same LOS, improve the quality outcomes

Although effective by the standards listed above, critical paths have understandable limitations that are still evident today. These limitations are only magnified if critical paths are used merely as a policing, audit mechanism rather than the clinical outcome-producing process emphasis from which they arose.

- Critical paths emphasize tasks or interventions, rather than outcomes.
- Critical paths cannot replace any specific documents in the permanent medical record. Although they do constitute a multidisciplinary action plan, they have no built-in evaluation of results.
- Variances from planned interventions listed on the critical path basically constitute a process audit, making clinicians wary of change processes (a necessary step in individualizing care) lest there be a variance.

Design #4. CareMap Tools

To address these deficits, critical paths were expanded to incorporate clinical progressions estimated against the planned time frame. These progressions constitute ongoing patient and family evaluation criteria, and are called intermediate goals and outcomes on the CareMap tool. The whole new section is sometimes referred to as the *Quality Index.*

CareMap tools are the newest breakthrough in cost/quality outcome management. They have evolved from their longer version, case management plans, and their condensed version, critical paths, into user-friendly documents that:

- Replace nursing care plans on patient care plans
- Describe the contributions of every department
- Show standards of care and standards of practice, and the timed, sequenced relationship between the two for a given case type, DRG, ICD-9 code, or constellation of problems
- Individualize care through analyzing and acting upon variances
- Give each discipline the opportunity to streamline documentation by charting by exception (variance), with the CareMap tool representing the "norm" (non-exception)
- Provide a database for CQI
- Integrate the acuity systems, costing systems, and research

CareMap tools are cause-and-effect grids; that is, staff actions should result in patient/family reactions or responses, which over time are "transformed" into desired outcomes. A sample grid for congestive heart failure is shown in figure 1-6.

CareMap tools are built on the basic formula shown in figure 1-7. This formula encompasses complex practice patterns, which themselves have many sources. To build a CareMap tool requires deep respect for the knowledge, concern, and tradition that clinicians in every discipline use in the care of patients. Practice patterns are based on research, experience, preference, convenience, ethics, regional influences, and other variables. They reflect good practice and can never replace good judgment.

Like their critical path predecessors, CareMap tools chart phenomena associated with a homogeneous patient population as demonstrated in figure 1-7 along two axes: action and time. Critical paths chart only multidisciplinary staff actions in terms of interventions against the time line most appropriate for the phase of treatment of a specific population. CareMap tools go a step further by including expected patient/family responses to staff interventions in terms of outcome criteria and intermediate measures of progress. Figure 1-8 diagrams the difference between a critical path and a CareMap tool.

Patient/family actions are categorized by problem statements that transform into intermediate goals and, by the last time frame, outcomes. These actions are measurable and behavioral, and may include responses in the categories of physiology, self-care, activities of daily living, follow-up plans, psychology, and absence of complications often related to patient medical diagnoses.

In 1987, Stetler and DeZell suggested four generic categories that should always be considered for inclusion in problem/outcome statements. These are:[7]

1. *Potential for complications of self-care:* Presence of risk factors that may limit a patient's ability to manage his or her own disease and/or engage in health-promoting activities in the home environment
2. *Potential for injury unrelated to treatment:* Presence of risk factors related primarily to the patient's general state of health and/or the specific disease symptom that could lead to physical injury within the institutional setting
3. *Potential for complications related to treatment:* Presence of risk factors (at times inherent in in-hospital treatment) that endanger the health and safety of the patient if appropriate preventive measures are not instituted and maintained and/or if ongoing observations and monitoring are not instituted
4. *Potential for extension of the disease process:* Presence of a specific condition or pathological process that carries with it a risk that endangers the patient's recovery—that is, presence of a risk that will be increased if a treatable extension or sequela are undetected

As the outcome management movement becomes more influential, new proposals for categories by which to define and measure positive outcomes will emerge. For

Figure 1-6. CareMap Tool Grid: Congestive Heart Failure

Location / Problem	Day 1 — ER 1–4 hours	Day 1 — Floor Telemetry or CCU 6–24 hours	Day 2 — Floor	Day 3 — Floor	Day 4 — Floor	Day 5 — Floor	Day 6 — Floor
				Benchmark Quality Criteria			
1) Alteration in gas exchange/profusion and fluid balance due to decreased cardiac output, excess fluid volume	Reduced pain from admission or pain free; Uses pain scale; O₂ sat. improved over admission baseline on O₂ therapy	Respirations equal to or less than on admission	O_2 sat = 90; Resp 20–22; Vital signs stable; Crackles at lung bases; Mild shortness of breath with activity	Does not require O_2; Vital signs stable; Crackles at base; Respirations 20–22; Mild shortness of breath with activity	Does not require O_2 (O_2 sat. on room air 90%); Vital signs stable; Crackles at base; Respirations 20–22; Completes activities with no increase in respirations; No edema	Can lie in bed at baseline position; Chest X-ray clear or at baseline	No dyspnea
2) Potential for shock	No signs/symptoms of shock	No signs/symptoms of shock	No signs/symptoms of shock	No signs/symptoms of shock; Normal lab values	No signs/symptoms of shock	No signs/symptoms of shock	No signs/symptoms of shock
3) Potential for consequences of immobility and decreased activity: skin breakdown, DVT	No redness at pressure points; No falls	No redness at pressure points; No falls	Tolerates chair, washing, eating, and toileting	Has bowel movement; Up in room and bathroom with assist	Up ad lib for short periods	Activity increased to level used at home without shortness of breath	Activity increased to level used at home without shortness of breath
4) Alteration in nutritional intake due to nausea and vomiting, labored		No c/o nausea; No vomiting; Taking liquids as offered	Eating solids; Takes in 50% each meal	Taking 50% each meal	Taking 50% each meal; Weight 2 lbs from patient's normal baseline	Taking 75% each meal	Taking 75% each meal
5) Potential for arrhythmias due to decreased cardiac output: decreased irritable foci, valve problems, decreased gas exchange	No evidence of life-threatening dysrhythmias	Normal sinus rhythm with benign ectopy	K(WNL); Benign or no arrhythmias	Digoxin level DNL; Benign or no arrhythmias	Digoxin level WNL; Benign or no arrhythmias	Digoxin level WNL; Benign or no arrhythmias	Digoxin level WNL; Benign or no arrhythmias
6) Patient/family response to future treatment & hospitalization	Patient/family expressing concerns; Following directions of staff	Patient/family expressing concerns; Following directions of staff	Patient/family expressing concerns; Following directions of staff	States reasons for and cooperates with rest periods; Patient begins to assess own knowledge and ability to care for CHF at home	Patient decides whether he/she wants discussion with physician about advanced directives	States plan for 1–2 days postdischarge as to meds, diet, activity, follow-up appointments; Expresses reaction to having CHF	Repeats plans; States signs and symptoms to notify physician/ER; Signs discharge consent
7) Individual problem							

Staff Tasks							
Assessments/Consults	Vital signs q 15 min Nursing assessments focus on lung sounds, edema, color, skin integrity, jugular vein distention Cardiac monitor Arterial line if needed Swan Ganz Intake & output	Vital signs q 15 min–1 hr Repeat nursing assessments Cardiac monitor Arterial line Swan Ganz Daily weight Intake & output	Vital signs q 4 hrs Repeat nursing assessments D/C cardiac monitor 24 hr D/C arterial and Swan Ganz Daily weight Intake & output	Vital signs q 6 hrs Repeat nursing assessments Daily weight Intake & output	Vital signs q 6 hrs Repeat nursing assessments Daily weight Intake & output Nutrition consult	Vital signs q 6 hrs Repeat nursing assessments Daily weight Intake & output	Vital signs q 6 hrs Repeat nursing assessments Daily weight Intake & output
Specimens/Tests	Consider TSH studies Chest X-ray EKG CPK q 8 hr x 3 ABG if pulse Ox: (range) Lytes, Na, K, Cl, CO_2 Glucose, BUN, Creatinine Digoxin: (range)	B/G	Evaluate for ECHO Lytes, BUN, Creatinine			Chest X-ray Lytes, BUN, Creatinine	
Treatments	O_2 or intubate IV or Heparin lock	O_2 IV or Heparin lock	IV or Heparin lock	DC pulse Ox if stable D/C IV or Heparin lock			
Medications	Evaluate for Digoxin Nitrodrip or paste Diuretics IV Evaluate for antiemetics Evaluate for antiarrhythmics	Evaluate for Digoxin Nitrodrip or paste Diuretics IV Evaluate for pre-load/after-load reducers K supplements Stool softeners	D/C Nitrodrip or paste Diuretics IV or PO K supplements Stool softeners Evaluate for nicotine patch	Change to PO Digoxin PO diuretics K supplements Stool softeners Nicotine patch if consent	PO diuretics K supplement Stool softeners Nicotine patch if consent	PO diuretics K supplement Stool softeners Nicotine patch if consent	PO diuretics K supplement Stool softeners Nicotine patch if consent
Nutrition	None	Clear liquids	Cardiac, low-salt diet	Cardiac, low-salt diet	Cardiac, low-salt diet	Cardiac, low-salt diet	
Safety/Activity	Commode Bedrest with head elevated Reposition patient q 2 hrs Bedrails up Call light available	Commode Bedrest with head elevated Dangle Reposition patient q 2 hrs Enforce rest periods Bedrails up Call light available	Commode Enforce rest periods Chair with assist ½ hr with feet elevated Bedrails up Call light available	Bathroom privileges Chair x 3 Bedrails up Call light available	Ambulate in hall x 2 Up ad lib between rest periods Bedrails up Call light available	Encourage ADLs that approximate activities at home Bedrails up Call light available	Encourage ADLs that approximate activities at home Bedrails up Call light available
Teaching	Explain procedures Teach chest pain scale and importance of reporting	Explain course, need for energy conservation Orient to unit and routine	Clarify CHF Dx and future teaching needs Orient to unit and routine Schedule rest periods Begin medication teaching	Importance of weighing self every day Provide smoking cessation information Review energy conservation schedule	Cardiac rehab level as indicated by consult Provide smoking cessation support Dietary teaching	Review CHF education material with patient	Reinforce CHF teaching
Transfer/Discharge Coordination	Assess home situation: notify significant other If no arrhythmias or chest pain, transfer to floor Otherwise transfer to ICU	Screen for discharge needs Transfer to floor	Consider Home Health Care referral		Evaluate needs for diet and anti-smoking classes Physician offers discussion opportunities for advanced directives	Appointment and arrangement for follow-up care with Home Health Care nurses Contact VNA	Reinforce follow-up appointments

Reprinted, with permission, from The Center for Case Management, South Natick, MA.

Figure 1-7. The CareMap Formula

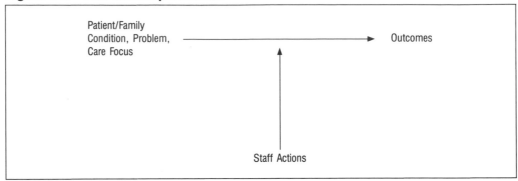

Figure 1-8. Problem/Outcome Index + Critical Path = CareMap Tool

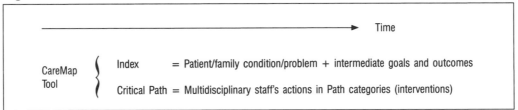

example, CareMap tool outcomes could be stated using "Short Form 36" categories such as well-being, functional status, and overall evaluation of health.[8] Positive measures such as these "afford a greater opportunity to integrate patients, providers, and payers. Such measures can be responsive to particular healthcare needs and goals, organizational capacity, technology, and economics."[9]

The challenge of having a precise but flexible tool that includes utilization review/appropriateness criteria, outcome criteria, and quality process criteria recorded concurrently is upon the industry. Developing not only concurrent tools but also those that require a single entry for each transaction after which the computer does the scheduling, linking, information sending, and tabulating is the work ahead.

A complete CareMap system includes variance analysis, use of an outcome–time focus in all multidisciplinary communication, case consultation and health care team meetings for patients at more-than-acceptable variance, and CQI. The challenge, of course, is to create a dynamic system of complex care management from a static piece of paper. This can be accomplished with a series of CareMap tools for different phases of treatment, the use of structured extensions or inserts, and the use of blank CareMap tools for anecdotal documentation or for those patients who require a totally individualized map. When a patient's reason for remaining in the hospital changes in a major way (for example, remaining on a vent after a craniotomy), the CareMap tool changes as well.

The ultimate result of a CareMap system is that unnecessary variance is reduced to a minimum because of an increasingly accurate learning curve that helps clinicians predict, prevent, and manage. It is not unusual for collaborative groups to begin developing CareMap documents for the more straightforward diagnoses, proceed to several varieties of that map, combine constellations of problems, and finally map care for the patient populations that were initially felt to be totally unpredictable.

Currently, CareMap tools are used either on paper as references only, on paper as permanent documentation, or on personal computers. As institutions and clinicians become comfortable with CareMap tool development, and as computer systems convert to CareMap systems, higher percentages of patients will be managed by them (with daily or per visit screens). Similarly, variances are presently being handled differently depending on each agency's goals for implementing the system in the first place. Minimally, patient/family and community variances are recorded in the medical record. A few institutions have decided to include clinician- and hospital-generated variances in the chart as well.

A CareMap system implies more than using a new document to manage care. At the heart of the system is vigilant attention to patient/family outcomes, with increasingly more authority used at the multidisciplinary clinical level. However, the tool is only as useful as the people on whose practices it is built.

As representatives from various disciplines try not to step on each other's toes, passivity and avoidance become so common that literally no decisions can be made. Sometimes disciplines either just do not know the right way to proceed with a patient whose condition is highly complex or do not have enough information to make a decision. Often the environment is one in which the different disciplines have tentative expectations of each other. The one major change in behavior required in a CareMap system is the shift from passive "care following" to proactive care management.[10] Proactive care management is directed toward agreed-on progressions of outcomes.

The shift to outcome-based practice as exemplified and guided by a CareMap system is subtle but profound. To be effective, the system must develop new avenues to discuss outcomes across care areas from acute care to wellness with patients/families. Education and monitoring must be in place that expect and evaluate the accountabilities of specific professional clinicians for defined outcomes.

Case Management

CareMap tools and other collaborative documents such as patient assessment forms, outcome tests, and so on address the what and, to some extent, the how of care. The depth of an automated system can further describe the why and how of care, based on extensive algorithms and policies. The who of care (the conductor or integrator of the many processes) is addressed by case management models.

Brief History

"Case management can simultaneously be described as a system, a role, a technology, a process, and a service."[11] In this text, it is referred to as a clinical system that focuses on the accountability of an identified individual or group for the following:

* Coordinating a patient's or group of patients' care across an episode or continuum of care
* Ensuring and facilitating the achievement of quality and clinical cost outcomes
* Negotiating, procuring, and coordinating services and resources needed by the patient/family
* Intervening at key points (and/or at significant variances) for individual patients
* With the collaborative teams, addressing and resolving patterns in aggregate variances that have a negative quality–cost impact
* Creating opportunities and systems to enhance outcomes

Case management is a paradoxically simple, yet complex concept. Its fundamental focus is to integrate, coordinate, and advocate for individuals, families, and groups requiring extensive services. The ultimate goal is to achieve planned care outcomes by brokering services across the health care continuum. Although case management may be directed toward other goals, and although the primary purpose for instituting a case management system may vary among programs, coordination of care is the basic component of all case management models and modalities. The term *case management* is generic, and modifiers are beginning to emerge to differentiate the various case management models.[12]

Case management exists within many contexts and settings. These include:

- Insurance-based programs
- Employer-based programs
- Workers' compensation programs
- Social services programs
- Independent practice
- Medical practice
- Nursing practice
- Public health nursing and Visiting Nurses Association practices
- Maternal and child health settings
- Mental health settings

Precursors to the advent of case management models in acute care were case management of frail elderly and handicapped children in the community, as well as the coordination of multiservices for transplant patients and people with AIDS. Managing patients between the hospital and home to follow up on discharge plans was begun at Carondelet St. Mary's Hospital in Tucson, Arizona.[13] Case management as a major restructuring of roles and systems for collaborative care was begun in 1986 at New England Medical Center Hospitals.

Case management was begun as a method to give selected primary staff nurses a larger scope of practice and span of control in providing patients and families better coordinated acute care within shorter time periods. In other words, the case manager used a process that created a classic "linking pin" function for all services, expediting care across time and setting. Although this new concept in acute health care made common sense, it went against traditional wisdom about the structure of jobs and health care organizations.

> Throughout the industrial age, the emphasis has been on seeking efficiencies through the detailed functional specialization of jobs or the so-called functional division of labor. Now, however, many firms are beginning to move toward combination, not division, of labor. They are using individuals or small teams to perform a series of tasks, such as the fulfillment of a customer order from beginning to end, often with the help of information systems that reach through the organization.[14]

The goal at NEMCH was not to add layers of case managers but, rather, to use primary nurse caregivers as case managers who would focus their direct patient care assignments on the specific patient populations of specific physicians. If the patient traveled to several units, a predetermined primary nurse on each unit would take over. These serially assigned primary nurses formed a nursing group practice paired with one or more attending-level physicians and joined by representatives from each key discipline in a formal collaborative care group. In this model, every collaborative care group had a case management plan and, eventually, a critical path as a shorthand guide. (CareMap systems were not yet available.)

Beginning in fall of 1987, a set of ground rules guided the continued implementation of case management. (See figure 1-9.) While maintaining their usual primary nursing and shift responsibilities, selected staff nurses entered the newly formed group practices by attending a three-day curriculum. They then began the awesome task of joining standards, management tools, and care delivery with each other and with those physicians whose patients they shared. The patient populations initially addressed were the catastrophically ill (for example, cardiology, stroke, oncology, vascular surgery, and

Figure 1-9. Case Management Ground Rules

- Every designated patient will be assigned to a nursing group practice on or before entry to the system.
- Every group practice will assign a nursing case manager who works with an attending physician in evaluating an individualized Case Management Plan (CMP) and Critical Path for each patient.
- A Critical Path is used to facilitate the care for every patient.
- Report will be based on Critical Paths.
- Negative variances from Critical Paths and/or CMPs require discussion with the attending physician, and a case management consultation when necessary.
- Every case manager must be a primary nurse or an associate when the patient is in his/her geographic area.
- The nursing case manager and physician case manager must communicate on a regular basis.
- Case managers will evolve/negotiate a flexible schedule that accommodates the needs of their patients and group practice as well as the needs of their units.
- Responsibility of the case manager begins at notification of patient's entry into the system and ends with a formal transfer of accountability to the patient, family, another health care provider or another institution.

so on), those requiring major resource utilization during most phases of their acute care. No additional nurses were added to the budget to accommodate this goal. Following is a description of how case management worked for patients at NEMCH:

If you are admitted for an abdominal aortic aneurysm repair, you become a patient of a collaborative practice composed of two vascular physicians and four staff nurses who treat you throughout your entire episode of care. In fact, you probably are already followed by the physicians and the ambulatory nurse member of the group practice. Now that you are entering acute care, she will notify her group of your special needs and work with the physician to facilitate a smooth pre-op course. The group uses the Critical Path for DRG 100-Major Vascular Surgery (10–13-day length of stay) to plan, track, and evaluate your progress.

When you arrive on the inpatient unit, the inpatient nurse in the group practice becomes either your primary nurse or associate primary nurse. She will discuss your Critical Path with you and your family and will help you become familiar with the sequencing of events. She will give you direct care before the OR and after your SICU stay.

She will also coordinate your transitions with the OR/RR nurse member of the group practice and with the nurse member from the SICU. In fact, she will meet you before surgery, offer to take you on a tour of the SICU, and answer any questions you or your family may have.

The group practice communicates often with your surgeon and meets formally for about an hour a week to discuss their 30 active patients. Although these nurses are part of the regular staffing on each of their units, they take vascular patients within their primary caseloads and shift assignments. When any one of them is not on duty, their peers on their own units continue to follow the Critical Path in a way similar to following a nursing care plan.

When you are ready for discharge, she will again meet with you to reinforce your followup appointments in the ambulatory setting. With the surgeon and the rest of the group practice, she will assess your achievement of the outcomes as well as analyze any variances from the Critical Path that you may have encountered. By doing this, they can better anticipate your future needs and can also improve the way our system works.

This first group practice demonstrated in several ways that "the whole is more than the sum of the parts." By viewing the whole episode of care as each of their responsibilities, they uncovered not only problems, but effective solutions. For instance several surgeries a week were being cancelled because patients who were already admitted and scheduled were not passing a Thallium-Persantine Scan (stress test). The group practice suggested that these scans as well as angiograms be done on an outpatient basis. They were able, through their nurse managers, to negotiate a set time for these scans, reserved by the vascular service. They then wrote a letter to patients explaining the importance of the scans and their scheduling. By this one change, they saved OR time, and eliminated unnecessary patient anxiety over surgery that might eventually not be performed. They have gained more control over their time and their environment.

Through enhanced communication between the nursing group and the physicians, they have cut SICU days from a range of 5–7 days to 3–5 days in the past year—without compromising standards. In addition, they have managed their caseload of patients through early intervention so well, that their patients (who tend to have complicated and chronic conditions with an estimated 70% on Medicare) do not frequent the Emergency Room.[15]

Eventually, ground rules for case management were formulated. In addition, each nursing group practice of staff nurse case managers was assisted to evolve group maintenance and development functions, including:

- Establishment of ongoing multidisciplinary collaborative practice groups who would strive for a unified philosophy and approach among nurses, physicians, all key disciplines, and patients and their families
- Revision of norms, values, and standards, stimulated by audits and research
- Entry and continuing education qualifications for case management nurses
- Peer review, quality assurance
- Peer consultation
- Time planning and shared benefits
- Case-based follow-up and research

The transition to case management and eventually to formal collaborative care groups for more than 20 patient populations was fostered by a spirit of experimentation and patient-centeredness. Although always room for improvement, there started to emerge "a new order of collaboration, one that was much more concrete and based on a clear understanding of expected patient care outcomes and the paths needed to reach them."[16]

Since that first application, numerous acute and home care organizations have used the rationale to design their own models. (See figure 1-10.) All the current case management models necessitate collaboration of some kind, but not all have inclusionary collaborative care as their overriding goal. (Chapter 8 elaborates on the design and use of dynamic case management models.)

Care Management versus Case Management

Care management is commonly confused with case management. Both strategies may use CareMap tools, but these terms represent two levels of care coordination. *Care management* is the provision of services to a patient in a distinct unit or area, whereas *case management* is the expedition of services across multiple care areas and, depending on the application, the procurement of health and prevention services beyond recuperation. Case management can be episodic, as in all services given to a client from first contact to last contact for a specific problem (chest pain through cardiac rehab) or continuum based (such as the maintenance of diabetes or handicaps throughout life). The entire acute and outpatient/homecare population receives care management. However, how that care is managed can be broken down into three categories. Figure 1-11 shows the relationship between case management, CareMap tools, and care delivery systems and suggests proportions of clients for whom the separate though related care coordination methods might be applied.

Care Management Models

Care management (also called care coordination) involves caregiver accountability at four levels of care: shift/visit, unit/department/discipline, episode, and continuum. (See figure 1-12.) At the shift and unit levels, the disciplines and departments (physicians, pharmacists, physical therapists, and so on) work with nursing to stabilize services in a variety of ways. Because the shift and unit levels have so many implications for

Figure 1-10. Case Management Rationale

Why Case Management?

1. Case management focuses on the full spectrum of needs presented by clients and their families; it is client-focused. Client and family satisfaction within case-managed systems is generally high.

2. A strong component of case management is an outcome orientation to care. The goal is to move with the client/family toward optimal care outcomes.

3. Case management facilitates and promotes coordination of client care, minimizing fragmentation.

4. Case management promotes cost-effective care by minimizing fragmentation, maximizing coordination, and facilitating client/family movement through the health care system.

5. Case management maximizes and coordinates the contributions of all disciplines within the health care team.

6. Case management responds to the needs of insurers and other third-party payers, specifically those related to outcome-based, cost-effective care.

7. The needs of clients, providers, and payers all receive attention within a case management system. Case management represents a merger of clinical and financial interests, systems, and outcomes.

8. Case management can be included in the marketing strategies of hospitals and other institutions to target clients/families, insurers, and employers.

Reprinted, with permission, from Bower, K. *Case Management by Nurses.* Washington, DC: The American Nurses' Association, 1992, pp. 7–8.

Figure 1-11. Recommended Percentages of Patients Covered by CareMap Tools, Care Management, and Case Management

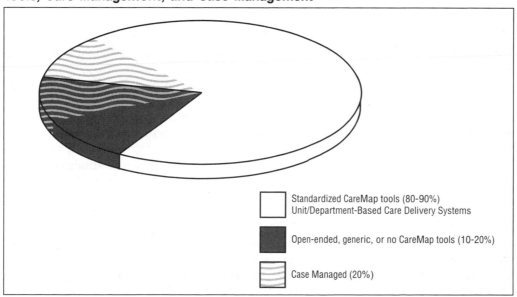

Standardized CareMap tools (80-90%)
Unit/Department-Based Care Delivery Systems

Open-ended, generic, or no CareMap tools (10-20%)

Case Managed (20%)

Figure 1-12. Expanding Scope of Accountability

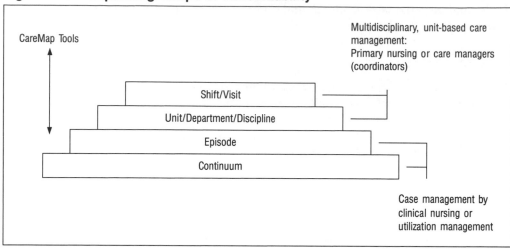

nurses, nursing must evaluate its internal, unit-based structure for accountability. The choices for nursing at the care delivery level are:

- No-accountability structure
- Primary nursing
- Care management

No-Accountability Structure

In this structure, care is organized by team, geography, function, or a "mixed" method, with no nurse actually managing a patient's care over time toward specific outcomes. Although the nurse manager is actually accountable, other responsibilities prevent him or her from fulfilling that expectation well. Thus, in these situations, accountability "defaults" to the physician, who traditionally is unavailable to attend to the myriad details required by each patient.

Primary Nursing

This is a solid accountability structure for the care delivery level. In fact, the CareMap tools and new collaborative attitudes make primary nursing easier to maintain. However, primary nursing is a "high-upkeep" model because every eligible nurse is expected to function with a vision and proactive energy for patients and families beyond his or her completion of tasks on a shift. This expectation requires a long-term commitment by nursing to constantly support the primary nursing model through weekly staff meetings and monthly primary nursing committee meetings, mandatory clinical management education for staff nurses beyond orientation, psychiatric liaison consultation for complicated care situations, nurse manager education for coaching and mentoring professional practice, and so on.

Primary nursing demands automatic assignments on or before admission and is not a layering method, although nurses may work with nonnursing staff. This model is a combined care delivery and accountability system.

Care Management

Care managers (coordinators) are a new option at the shift and unit levels. They function similarly to primary nurses but are fewer in number (generally, one to six per unit); and the care management model does not require the same level of support from managers and administrators as the primary nursing model does. Care managers may be assigned by unit district but more often are assigned by case type, physician, or some other definer.

Care managers might be budgeted as part of staffing and over several years be taken out of staffing numbers. Although this can create new problems, it also can create new opportunities. For example, a gerontology care manager tied to direct care patient assignments may not have the opportunity to always participate in corporate planning meetings for new gerontology programs because his or her first commitment is to take care of patients. When staffing is low, meetings and other chances to collaborate are low priority. When the care manager can attend, the agency benefits from the expert knowledge but the care unit perceives it as a temporary loss of manpower. When care managers are removed from the staffing budget, they have more flexibility.

Case Management Models

As health care organizations consider case management methods for the episode and continuum levels, they enter a political arena. Because case management is *not* a care delivery system, its design should not be determined exclusively by one department. In fact, there are many ways to structure accountability via case management. These include:

- *Case management by clinical nursing:* For example, exemplary primary nurses from serial or cluster units can be combined into formal nursing group practices that serve as a core of a case-type-specific collaborative practice group; or RNs who are either on the top clinical ladder step or already clinical specialists can be used to focus on a specific patient population and service.
- *Case management by utilization review (UR):* UR can have a combined UR–discharge planning function and serve more patients than those on one unit; or UR can be used as auditors of care processes and patient placement, as well as information specialists. In the latter example, UR staff function as adjuncts to managers, as well as collaborative groups at the product line or corporate CQI level of the organization.

The clinical nursing and UR models of case management have very different assumptions underlying their use, although they look somewhat the same on the surface. Both models have management of the cost-per-case budget as a major responsibility. How the cost, as well as clinical outcomes per case, are actually negotiated within a network of services will be different between UR and clinical nursing. (New structures to integrate these two case management approaches are discussed in chapter 10.)

The Relationship of Collaborative Care to Major Industry Trends

As can be seen from the evolution of collaborative care strategies, their continuous development is driven by finding the balance between cost, process, and outcome. Critical paths/CareMap systems and case management were *purposely* positioned so that they would force the discovery and operationalization of such a balance. Therefore, these two effective strategies by definition and design have a relationship to any trend in the industry. Their primary relationships are to:

- Finance/market contracts
- Continuous quality improvement
- Changes in physician practice
- Patient-focused care

25

Automated information systems and product line management are discussed in chapter 10.

Finance/Market Contracts

Although financial information has become more sophisticated and accessible since implementation of case management plans (CMPs), its basic principles have not changed. Precipitated by DRGs for Medicare patients, LOS became the number-one financial issue for acute care, followed by resources used within a LOS. In effect, the CMPs, followed by critical paths and CareMap tools, became written tables of planned resource consumption.

Indeed, if the true cost of every intervention by every discipline were known, a CareMap tool would accurately and comprehensively describe the planned cost per case type. Unfortunately, true costs for all disciplines have not yet been aggregated or tracked per case type, so at this time administrators and clinicians are dealing with representative costs.

Any group attempting to anticipate or evaluate the impact of collaborative care must consider certain general factors. These are:

1. *Physicians are not the sole culprits in cost or quality issues.* Although they have the lead role in ordering actions of other professionals and departments, orders are generated by patient need as determined by other disciplines as well as by physicians. For example, nursing staff may detect unclear urine necessitating an order for a culture and sensitivity test, or physical therapy may determine a need for a specific brace. The American system positions the physician as the one who must approve these requests, but it is important for collaborative care as well as for accurate financial planning to realize that physicians do not initiate all care needs.
2. *Cost-per-case automated systems have been built from costs generated by physicians' orders and not by the direct costs of other resources.* At present, these interventions (such as teaching by nurses, support by in-house clergy, or consultation by continuing care) are understood as part of overhead costs, which also are being examined. Clearly, the interventions of all disciplines per case type need to be calculated in order to determine accurate cost per case.

    Collaborative care is interdependent because each discipline responds to different phenomena in the mind and body of the recipients of that care. To estimate, manage, and measure true costs of resources, it is important to acknowledge that overall patient needs drive the costs and that each discipline, including the physicians, interprets those different needs to the larger caregiving organization.
3. *Data alone do not change practice.* Although data on LOS, mortality, infection, and readmission rates, for example, do draw attention, depending on the content and accuracy of the data, their display may actually alienate the very people who need to collaborate.

    In collaborative care, data on practice patterns are crucial to planning new ways of accomplishing tasks and achieving patient/family outcomes. Multidisciplinary groups need data on every aspect of cost and quality available. They need to review the data together to really understand the ramification of the data and to develop ideas about causality and change.
4. *Intensity of care usually increases as LOS decreases.* This is especially true if the clinical outcomes to be achieved do not change. Although only one published report justifies this statement, it makes sense intuitively.[17]
5. *LOS cannot be cut conscientiously without responding to cost and quality implications across an entire episode of care.* If patients having transurethral

prostatectomies, for example, are discharged by three days postop instead of five, their urine may be tainted with a little blood or small clots. They may feel weaker than they would have had they been discharged at five days. To be professionally responsible to such patients, any agency or payer changing LOS practices has to develop a system for the potential gaps in care delivery.

6. *Desired practice changes in regard to LOS require a continual focus or else old habits will creep back into behavior.* In addition, revised sequencing of staff activities and departmental support entail constant vigilance and monitoring on the part of managers and administrators. Getting a new program going is often easier than keeping it going over time!

Ultimately, knowing the cost per case is essential to sound negotiations for managed care contracts. Presently, however, negotiations are occurring without the benefit of complete information. Therefore, both acute and home care organizations that understand their future existence may depend on managed care contracts are using critical paths/CareMap systems and case management to firm up their internal structures and external credibility to produce desired outcomes.

One such institution is ScrippsHealth, part of the Scripps Institutions of Medicine and Science, a not-for-profit health care system in San Diego County, California. In response to doing a high percentage of global fee and managed care work, the principal group of cardiothoracic surgeons asked hospital administration to develop a case management model as a way to ensure that patients and their families would receive adequate education about their treatment. They developed CareTrac™, a version of CareMap tools for coronary artery bypass graft (CABG) and other case types.[18-20]

ScrippsHealth has had clinical, administrative, and financial success with its CareTracs™. In the past, hospitals and physicians were not at financial risk with each other (one group could make a profit while the other did not). Under global fee contracts, however, they are. Sharon Andersson, administrative director of quality resource management, reports that she must prepare information for negotiating market contracts in regard to whether they (1) have critical paths in place, (2) identify opportunities for improvement, and (3) are willing to share variance data. She also reports that third parties are pleased with the defined LOS, uniform outcomes, and facilitation of discharge planning created by the CareTracs™.

The home care industry is similarly preparing for managed care contracts reinforced by an internal CareMap system and case management approach. Following is the rationale for this approach:

The implementation of such managed care systems in home care agencies will enable the tracking of resource use by case type, in turn providing agencies with cost data that will allow them to better control those costs and predict profit or loss by each case type. Identification of costs by case type can further enhance an agency's ability to negotiate with third-party payers, health maintenance organizations, and preferred provider organizations.[21]

Continuous Quality Improvement

CareMap tools specifically operationalize continuous quality improvement (CQI). They do this through a distinct process that goes beyond the multidisciplinary authoring of the tools to their actual use in practice to the retrospective use of variance data. Any time clinical experts and the supporting departments formally define their processes and evaluate those desired processes and outcomes against actual events, continuous quality improvement is occurring.

Critical paths or a CareMap system, and when needed, case management, operationalize CQI where it matters most—at the direct patient care level. Critical paths/

CareMap tools describe the clinical work of each professional discipline and department as it relates to patient/family measurable outcomes of care. As mentioned previously, these outcomes are the quality standard toward which all other processes and interventions should be directed. When patient care is planned, given, documented, and evaluated using critical paths/CareMap tools around the clock, a reliable, tangible, dynamic CQI process is actualized. For example:

- Quality can be defined.
- The patient/family problem outcome method gives caregivers the ability to define and measure quality.
- The LOS time frame of a CareMap tool forces caregivers to pin down outcomes and then benchmark intermediate goals for an episode of care.
- Building a CareMap between clinical experts of all disciplines and departments related to specific patient populations creates a tangible definition of quality for everyone.
- The more an institution's experts can define expected results of their interventions for similar groups of patients, the better managers and administrators can support them.
- The more tightly quality is defined, the more need arises for the clear assignment of accountability.

Unless outcomes are defined, managed, and evaluated at the detailed patient–clinician level, there is no quality for the patient currently recurring, for quality entails precision of interventions as measured by their results. In a CareMap system, the desired end (outcome) does not justify all the means, but it does drive the means.

CareMap tools go beyond traditional critical paths because they include an "index" along the same timed axis as the interventions. With its problem–outcome statements, the index is the *quality descriptor.* In contrast, the critical path describes key interventions agreed on by clinical experts as fundamental to producing the outcomes. Thus, the critical path is the *cost descriptor.* A CareMap tool puts cost and quality in balance by combining the index with the critical path.

When a CareMap tool is used around the clock by each professional coming in contact with the patient, care management toward outcomes is tightly structured. The caregiver compares the patient's current status against that which is outlined in the index. Completed interventions and intermediate goals are signed off by the appropriate discipline. Different or unexpected interventions and goals are recorded according to each institution's documentation policies. These unexpected events are considered variances or exceptions, and often create a need for further action by the clinician.

Variances show where the CareMap plan differs from reality, which may be explained as positive or negative occurrences. Either way, variances are cause for analysis at the moment, and also provide an invaluable database for CQI when aggregated.

For a health care institution to truly know and address its quality issues, it must first define quality not as a process but as a product. When designed and used by all disciplines, a CareMap tool is the best method by which to accomplish not only the setting of standards but also the implementation and evaluation of those standards around the clock.

The CareMap as a Multidisciplinary Tool

A CareMap tool is only a piece of paper or a screen on a computer unless it becomes a tool for the actual micromanagement of the care it indicates. Progress can be made in true collaborative practice when there is:

1. Agreement about the expected clinical outcomes of interventions (which should be added to critical paths to make CareMap tools)
2. Determination made as to which clinical departments have authority to validate outcome achievement

CareMap tools should be multidisciplinary in every way. The ultimate goal is that professionals of each discipline who give direct care evaluate the patient and/or family against the intermediate outcomes every day, shift, hour, or visit. When used for documentation, CareMap tools have the potential of replacing progress notes for all disciplines unless there are variances, in which case a progress note is required by the discipline(s) determined best qualified to evaluate that outcome. Otherwise, the professionals authorized to sign off outcomes can put their initials on the actual CareMap document and enter a signature log on the back.

The following checklist can be used to evaluate the extent of multidisciplinary collaboration in a CareMap system. All related disciplines and departments should be actively involved in the following activities:

- Serving on the steering committee
- Determining case types
- Creating CareMap tools
- Determining validity/reliability from literature review
- Meeting professional/state standards
- Setting thresholds for variance
- Orienting peers to CareMap process
- Signing off tasks and/or outcomes
- Determining variance coding
- Concurrently revising CareMap tools
- Keeping progress notes for patient/family variances
- Participating in ongoing "expert groups" (the original author teams) to maintain CQI
- Developing and teaching case type management
- Conducting research

The following section presents an example of how multidisciplinary collaboration works with one case type in one institution.

Anticipated Recovery Paths

Chronic obstructive pulmonary disease (COPD) is one of the most difficult case types to "map" and manage. Patients with COPD challenge their caregivers to constantly assess and revise how staff interventions add up to realistic results. The Mercy and Unity Hospitals (now part of the Allina Health System in Minneapolis) call their CareMap tools anticipated recovery paths (ARPs) and use them to better coordinate collaborative care toward outcomes for their COPD population.[22]

ARP development is focused on diagnoses that are high volume, high cost, and/or high risk. COPD fits the bill on all accounts:

- *High volume:* Last year, there were 721 admissions, either primary or secondary, at Mercy and 479 at Unity.
- *High cost:* Costs can skyrocket if patients have respiratory failure, end up on a ventilator, and are in the ICU for a prolonged time period.
- *High risk:* With a chronic illness, many patients are elderly and at risk for frequent admissions and readmissions.

COPD resides in many different hospital units and receives care from many different physician types. Thus, it is an excellent case type for development of a more coordinated, consistent approach to patient care delivery.

Generally, five factors influence LOS for all patients with chronic diseases. These are:

1. Mental health and attitude
2. Support network of family or friends
3. Good nutritional status
4. Pain or other stress factors
5. Lack of activity causing deconditioning

The preceding factors must be considered in attempts to define and meet the goals for pulmonary rehabilitation. These goals are:

- To improve the patient's and concerned others' understanding and acceptance of his or her disease
- To promote endurance, strength, and independence
- To provide patients/families with knowledge of the support available
- To promote a meaningful and productive life-style by returning the patient to the highest-level functioning possible

These goals will all be met by an interdisciplinary team approach.

An interdisciplinary team approach enables patients to benefit from the experience and expertise of many disciplines in a coordinated and efficient manner. All evaluations and activities (such as ambulation, activities of daily living, low-level endurance exercises, and so on) will encourage patients to take control of their illness.

The new ARP for COPD provides awareness for the "extras" that disciplines such as respiratory therapy, occupational therapy, and social services (comprising the Pulmonary Rehabilitation Team) can provide to help improve outcome and potentially decrease readmissions.

For example, use of the ARP reminds the patient care team that, in addition to routine treatments, respiratory services can evaluate the need for oxygen both in the hospital and at home, evaluate the optimal use of metered dose inhalers (MDIs), teach breathing techniques and effective coughing, and perform caloric needs assessment via indirect calorimetry (IDC).

Likewise, occupational therapy plays a key role in the interdisciplinary team approach because it is of great assistance in teaching daily living and coping skills. Sessions in improving tolerance to exercise/exertion, reinforcing correct breathing patterns, and learning self-relaxation techniques help to minimize patient breathing problems in the hospital and after discharge. Making the patient aware of energy-saving tips and body mechanics can make a critical difference in maintaining life-style and a positive outlook on life.

Social services contributes to the interdisciplinary team by planning the most effective use of care and resources. The social worker works with the patient with COPD and his or her family to help them cope with various effects of the disease such as anxiety, role changes, and financial concerns.

The Pulmonary Rehabilitation Team has been incorporated into the COPD ARP, and can be conveniently ordered by requesting Pulmonary Rehab Team or by checking "yes" and signing the pulmonary rehab sticker on the patient's order sheet.

To reinforce the collaborative management of high-quality care, several institutions have begun to include introductory classes about CareMap systems in their hospital orientation sessions. They also have rewritten each department's policies/procedures/responsibilities in relation to using the CareMap tool.

Dr. Donald Berwick, renowned for his leadership in quality improvement in health care, states that patients "need a system but get 'events.'"[23] The COPD example shows how management of high-quality care measured by outcomes using a CareMap tool is the foundation of "systemness."

The Use of Variances in the CareMap System

Just as CareMap tools are the heart of collaboratively managing care toward cost and quality outcomes, variances are the soul of a CareMap system. As mentioned earlier, variances show how and why clinicians and patients differ from the norm, as well as where an institution might improve on its service. A CareMap document without the variance component is a process without evaluation.

Although at face value the term *variance* is a simple idea meaning "exception" or "difference," formal variance can occur only when there is an established norm or standard. All clinicians use what is deemed "normal" in domains such as chemistry, anatomy, and psychology throughout their professional careers, as well as compare actual patients against that normal measure. The comparison, usually termed *assessment*, leads to a series of interventions designed to adjust or correct the variance if it is causing real or potential problems for the patient.

A CareMap system formalizes the norms in a number of ways. For example, it:

- Provides a written description of patient problems, intermediate goals, outcomes, and staff interventions validated among experts of all related professions.
- Establishes thresholds of time periods (hour, day, visit, week) within which the phenomenon described above should occur.
- Establishes 100 percent thresholds in terms of:
  - Either this intermediate goal or outcome was met as described, or it was not.
  - Either this staff intervention occurred as described, or it did not.
  - If not, a variance is considered to be present.

In a CareMap system, variances become more visible than they do in less-structured clinical methods. The CareMap system is designed to have clinicians caring for each patient ask themselves these questions:

- What should we be doing? How should the results of our work with patients and their families be observed?
- What actually is happening, and is there a variance?
- What is causing the variance?
- What do we need to do about it?
- How do we record variances for specific patients and for CQI data?

In effect, these questions are the scientific method operationalized at the caregiver level. In other words, they are the classic helping process, and variance analysis structures the evaluation step. Put simply:

The purpose of identifying variances is to evaluate what works and what needs refinement. It is not only essential to identify when a variance occurs but to hypothesize why the variance occurred in order that corrective actions can be implemented. Each variance and subsequent corrective action is evaluated for effectiveness by the clinicians. This early identification and immediate correction of variances is crucial to managing care for individual patients.[24]

Of most interest recently, the use of variance extends the scientific method used concurrently with each individual patient to the level of CQI by providing the quantitative information needed for collaborative practice groups to evaluate the effects of care for groups of their own patients in similar case types. Figure 1-13 compares the generic steps in clinical decision making between the scientific method, the CareMap system, and the CQI technique.

A question that has begun to emerge is: Do we really have to have a variance data system in order to continue to learn from our practice, to change, and to grow professionally? Sometimes the problems seem so obvious that clinicians have little tolerance for a data system that often demonstrates what they already believe they know!

But knowing is different from learning, and helping "smart people learn"[25] is the challenge of a CareMap system that uses variance data. At the individual patient level, this is clinical inquiry. To look at trends and interrelationships in groups of patients is taking clinical inquiry to another level of endeavor.

Changes in Physician Practice

Contrary to the much-too-prevalent opinion, physicians are not the adversaries to cost-effectiveness, quality, or other positive changes that hospitals are trying to accomplish. In fact, the less physicians are stereotyped, the less resistance they will offer, individually or as a group. Like everyone else, physicians are part of a highly interdependent system and will not change unless behaviors in other sectors of the system change as well.

Physicians need excellent hospitals and home care services to treat their patients; in turn, those agencies need excellent physicians. Increasingly, no group is immune from society's trust that health care will be provided with a responsibility to cost-effectiveness and quality. Simply put, if either physicians or health care institutions are at financial risk or cannot meet the array of regulations and accreditation standards, both parties cannot continue their mission.

Because changes in society and finances require physicians and institutions to be more collaborative, changes must occur within the context of physicians' high value on autonomy and individuality. Berwick comments that "... physicians seem to have

Figure 1-13. Effects of CareMap Systems and Collaborative Care on Physician Practice

- Patients express higher levels of satisfaction.
- Increases the likelihood that patients will receive the care desired no matter where they are in the institution or whether the nurse for that shift is "part-time." Keeps all other care providers "in synch" with the physician's plan of care.
- The physician retains control over patient care. Those activities which currently require a physician's order continue to do so. Physicians are actively involved in the development of Critical Paths or CareMap tools, reflecting the care they have determined their patients need.
- Reduces the need for involvement by Utilization Review.
- Provides a group of staff nurses and potentially other members of the healthcare team who are interested in and committed to the physician's practice case types. (Collaborative Care, Case Management)
- Facilitates the resolution of system issues that are often annoying and/or frustrating to the physician.
- The time requirement of the physician for the system is minimal (about 1–2 hours for CareMap development).
- Communication between the physician and the nurses is improved. Collegiality is strengthened.
- In some cases can enhance physician's revenue by reducing "lost" OR time, etc.
- Decreases the number of phone calls to the physician's office.
- In some areas, can be used in negotiations with PPOs or HMOs by physicians.
- Allow research findings to be readily incorporated into practice.

difficulty seeing themselves as participants in processes, rather than as lone agents of success or failure."[26]

Hospitals can only stay financially viable and improve just so far without at least some involvement from the physicians who use their services. The patient is the common denominator, the shared territory, the reason for existence. And since the advent of DRGs and other reimbursement limits, patient case types and resources used within an LOS have become the new definition for financial and quality viability between physicians and hospitals.

As a result, case type is the new common language of physicians and hospitals. Determining a best-production process from diagnosis through treatment to achieve measurable, detailed clinical outcomes is the new point of collaboration. These case type–specific outcomes are the tangible measure of quality. Berwick states that quality improvement "has little chance of success in health care organizations without the understanding, participation, and in many cases the leadership of individual doctors. In hospitals, physicians both rely on and help shape almost every process pertaining to a patient's experience, from support services (such as dietary and housekeeping functions) to clinical care services (such as laboratories and nursing). Few can improve without the help of medical staff."[27]

Five years ago, many physicians did not seem motivated to find a cost–quality balance. As with nurses and other health care professionals, they did not generally believe that the terms *cost-effectiveness* and *quality* belonged in the same sentence. In fact, physicians saw cost and quality as mutually exclusive.

A number of studies show that physicians were unaware of the costs of various categories of care.[28-30] Even those who were aware were understandably irritated and defensive if pressured by insurers, hospitals, and other groups to review and perhaps revise their ordering of medications, tests, consults, and related practices. Managed care and case management, when imposed externally to care providers, were perceived by physicians as financial policing actions with little attention paid to the quality of care.

Physicians care most about accurately diagnosing and treating *their* patients, using whatever resources necessary. They assume that quality will follow accuracy and that quality improvements not related to accurate orders will be addressed by the hospital. Many physicians do not like to be "bothered" with problems perceived to be extraneous to their immediate practice.

Traditionally, cost and quality have been separated in professional education and clinical information systems. The problem has been compounded because hospitals began computerizing their financial systems before their clinical records. Often the result is a system that attempts to merge pieces of clinical and financial information but leaves much to be desired. For example, *quality* is still defined broadly as mortality, morbidity, readmission, and infection rates, offering little new information to physicians. Costs per physician can be aggregated and reviewed in terms of LOS and orders generated, but the resulting data leave many physicians cold.

When critical paths, CareMap systems, and collaborative care models were introduced as a way to reflect and coordinate *individual physician preference* within the care provider institution, physicians became more intrigued with determining a cost–quality balance. Due to multiple, complex, and seemingly daily changes in the reimbursement and regulatory arenas, physicians are increasingly motivated to work with institutions—their administrators and clinicians—to implement new clinical systems that might achieve cost–quality outcomes for all concerned. Figure 1-14 gives 12 potential effects of a CareMap system and collaborative care models, sometimes referred to as case management. Clinical economics, outcomes management, and CQI are all collaborative processes that, when tied to a CareMap system, promote physician attention to both cost and quality.

Physicians can be engaged in a brief discussion about both their preferences and discharge criteria for a specific patient population. They tend to be very precise about intermediate and final outcome parameters, referred to by one chief of obstetrics and gynecology as "clinical indicators along a time line." However, when the discussion is formalized on paper, some physicians tend to be wary despite the trend toward guidelines.[31] Most of their hesitation stems from their concern about the ultimate uses of the paper document.

Thus, a plan for evolving a CareMap system needs to be developed between hospital and physicians. These questions will need answers:

- Are these standing orders?
- What happens if I don't follow the CareMap tool?
- What happens when the patient doesn't follow the CareMap tool?
- Who will review the CareMap tool?
- How will variances be analyzed and documented?
- How will the institution and insurers use the information?
- Am I more suable because of a CareMap tool?

Even when these questions are resolved, some physicians will not believe that certain case types are "mappable," and even if they believe treatment of a case type is somewhat predictable, they will not want their practice on paper, regardless of the number of examples they see from other institutions. Often such physicians are concerned that they will be subject to more intensive peer review and public scrutiny than they are currently. Clearly, these physicians will not be eager to be involved in CareMapping until either their concerns are addressed or they feel a greater threat from another sector of the industry that converts CareMap systems into perceived salvation.

As mentioned previously, CareMap systems require around-the-clock attention by all disciplines. They create a new level of accountability and pressure, often bringing to light direct care delivery issues such as problematic physician management practices. Although the issues that emerge usually are no surprise, the CareMap system, especially when it is part of a commitment to CQI, highlights the demand for resolution. Likewise, many institutional policies that aggravate physicians also become subject to resolution.

Figure 1-14. Comparison of Generic Steps in Clinical Decision Making

	Scientific Method	CareMap System Concurrent Use	CareMap System Retrospective Use	CQI Technique (PDCA)
1.	Assess	Assess		
2.	Plan; using problem/ approach statements	Plan; using a CareMap tool with collaboratively determined outcome measures	CareMap tool	Plan
3.	Intervene	Intervene		Do
4.	Evaluate	Evaluate; using variance Compare Consult Analyze Document	Aggregate Variance	Check
5.			Inform Discuss Revise CareMap if needed Make other changes	Act

Source: PDCA Control circle from Ishikawa, K. *What Is Total Quality Control? The Japanese Way*. Englewood Cliffs: Prentice-Hall, Inc., 1985, 59.

Collaboration is a loaded term and seems to mean more to nonphysicians than to physicians. The problem lies in the interpretation of the term. It may mean anything from getting a physician to respond to a page or a request to getting the physician's respect as a fellow colleague. Nonphysicians look for behavioral indications on the part of physicians, and often interpret "spending time" and "giving attention" as collaborative activities.

An unspoken acknowledgment of interdependence and demonstrated mutual respect is the principal building block of collaboration not only in nurse–physician relationships but in all effective working relationships. One panel of clinicians judged by peers as highly collaborative listed the building blocks of collaboration as: ". . . clinical expertise, consistency, credibility, assertive style, and formal structure for communication."[32]

For some physicians, it is eye-opening to realize how much effort nurses and others make in actualizing orders, as well as in responding to patient/family needs that are not a result of orders. Often they come to appreciate the value of genuine teamwork and believe they and their patients will directly benefit from it. While director of medical liaison at Scripps Memorial Hospitals in San Diego, Dr. Bruce Campbell gave the following advice:

> It is important to inform physicians that Critical Paths are not just an efficiency mechanism, but that they increase quality as well. In addition, Critical Paths are also a good communication tool. Involve physicians in the creation of the document from the beginning and explain that you will need their input periodically because Critical Paths are not a static phenomenon—they need continuous change and updating.
>
> Critical Paths are not cookbooks because they are not used to limit care. They fit a range of 30–70% of the population, and are minimum standards for all patients of that same population; Critical Paths specify the essential components of care for every patient with a given diagnosis.
>
> Care is so complex now, and variable from patient to patient, that if the essential components of care are not "blueprinted" they are either forgotten or not done on time. As a result, patient outcomes are jeopardized.
>
> Critical Paths appeal to the scientific method that physicians follow. They can be an *applied research process*. Clinical algorithms can be imbedded in the Critical Path; i.e., algorithms for whether a stroke patient should receive subcutaneous heparin for potential DVT (Deep Vein Thrombosis). For example, Scripps has included a swallow evaluation by RNs in their Critical Paths for stroke patients with space to document results which, in turn, trigger new actions. Finally, outcomes should be attached to the processes on a Critical Path [thus creating a CareMap tool] and results should be reviewed not per individual physician but per system. This encourages physicians' involvement in continuous quality improvement.[33]

Patient-Focused Care

Patient-focused care (PFC) is a set of principles and strategies that contribute to the appropriate restructuring of an organization. Following is a summation of these principles:[34]

- Resources must focus on the needs of patients and physicians.
- Services must be highly responsive to customer demands.
- Staff must be empowered in their pursuit of excellence.
- Continuity of care must be maintained to the fullest extent.
- Functions and processes must be efficient and effective.

The strategies for restructuring begin with fact gathering, patient grouping, and service delivery revision; then proceed to operational redesign, including operating policies and procedures; and end with restructuring enablers and performance targets.[35] Certainly collaborative care includes the same principles as PFC, although collaborative care is conceptualized with the patient/family clinical measurable outcomes as the basis of an organization's and an individual professional's contract with society. In other words, the needs of patients and their families are superordinate to the needs of the professionals. In collaborative care, continuity and efficiency of care services are means to effectiveness; in other words, did all those processes lead to precise, desired outcomes?

Collaborative care is at the level of "service delivery approach" in the PFC care model of restructuring. Fact finding, patient grouping, and critical paths/CareMap tools aid in restructuring and reinforcing new service delivery approaches—for example, the use of case managers to coordinate care across multiple service areas. The success of collaborative care will necessitate the PFC strategies of operational redesign, operating policies, and motivators for desired changes in performance. These are sound methods from the organizational development field.

Conclusion

In recent years, the concept of collaborative care has gained impetus in the health care industry as demands have increased for greater financial effectiveness through efforts such as decreased hospital length of stay and increased resource utilization. The concept is based on the idea that all caregiver activities are interdependent and that a concentrated collaborative effort on the part of all of a patient's caregivers will focus on priorities and solutions that will move his or her care toward optimal outcomes.

Among the formal mechanisms devised to make collaborative care a reality, critical paths and their second generation, CareMap tools, and case management have been demonstrated to be successful. Work completed by the nursing staff at New England Medical Center Hospitals (NEMCH) in Boston has focused on establishing the conceptual link between cost, process, and outcome. Four designs for planning, managing, documenting, and evaluating multidisciplinary care toward outcomes emerged: case management plans, time lines, critical paths, and CareMap tools.

Case management is often confused with care management. *Case management* is a structure in which care is planned by brokering services across the care continuum, extending from unit to unit and into the patient's life-style. *Care management* is the coordination of care within a specific unit or area. Both case management and care management are accomplished through a number of management models.

Critical paths/CareMap tools and case management were designed to work with any trend within the health care industry, including finance/market contracts, continuous quality improvement, changes in physician practice, and patient-focused care, always moving toward solidifying the link between cost, process, and outcome. As the industry grapples with the impact of collaborative care and begins to negotiate managed care contracts, two major obstacles must be overcome: (1) As a group, physicians have tended to resist managed care, first, as an infringement on their decision-making authority and, second, as an attempt to curb cost at the expense of quality of care; and (2) the true costs of all interventions in all disciplines are not known. However, in many cases the use of the different collaborative care strategies are converting physicians and helping to identify costs. For example, cardiac physicians at ScrippsHealth in San Diego County, California, asked their administration to develop a case management model to educate patients about their care. The model, called CareTrac™, has proved successful.

Collaborative care enables patients to benefit from the experience and expertise of an interdisciplinary team working together to manage their care in a coordinated and cost-effective manner. The goal is to contain cost and improve outcome without interfering with the process or quality of care. It is a goal that physicians, nonphysicians, patients, and families alike can embrace.

References

1. National Joint Practice Commission. *Guidelines for Establishing Joint or Collaborative Practice Hospitals.* Chicago: NJPC, 1981.

2. Zander, K. Revising the production process: when "more" is not the solution. *The Healthcare Supervisor* 3(3):44–54, Apr. 1985.

3. DeZell, A. D. Case management plans: a collaborative model. *Definition* 2(1):1–4, Winter 1987.

4. Zander, K. Timelines: the maps for managed care. *Definition* 1(3):1–3, Fall 1986.

5. Woldum, K. Critical paths: making the course. *Definition* 2(3):1–4, Summer 1987.

6. Zander, K., Etheredge, M. L., and Bower, K. *Nursing Case Management: Blueprints for Transformation.* Boston: New England Medical Center Hospitals, 1987, pp. 97–109.

7. Stetler, C., and DeZell, A. D. *Case Management Plans: Designs for Transformation.* Boston: Center for Nursing Case Management, New England Medical Center Hospitals, 1987.

8. Ellwood, P. M., and others. *The Future: Clinical Outcomes Management in Health Care Quality Management for the 21st Century.* Tampa, FL: ACPE Press, 1991

9. Geehr, E. The search for what works. *Healthcare Forum Journal* 34(4):28–31, July/Aug. 1992.

10. Zander, K. Responsive restructuring: turning care following into care management. *The New Definition* 9(1):1–3, Winter 1994.

11. Bower, K. *Case Management by Nurses.* Washington, DC: American Nurses' Association, 1992, pp. 2–7.

12. Bower.

13. Rusch, S. Continuity of care: from hospital unit into home. *Nursing Management* 17(12):31–41, 1986.

14. Davenport, T., and Nohria, N. Case management and the integration of labor. *Sloan Management Review* 35(2):11, Winter 1994.

15. Zander, K. Nursing practice: the Cadillac in continuity. *Definition* 3(2):1–2, Spring 1988.

16. Bower, K. Case management: meeting the challenge. *Definition* 3(1):3, Winter 1988.

17. Cohen, E. Nursing case management: does it pay? *Journal of Nursing Administration* 21(4):20–25, Apr. 1991.

18. Andersson, S. ScrippsHealth: quality planning for clinical processes of care. *The Quality Letter for Healthcare Leaders* 5(5):2–4, June 1993.

19. Campbell, A. B., and Lakier, N. CareTrac for cardiac patients. *Outcomes Measurement and Management,* Jan.–Feb. 1993, pp. 7–8.

20. Trubo, R. If this is cookbook medicine, you may like it. *Medical Economics* 70(6):69–82, Mar. 22, 1993.

21. Maturen, V., and Zander, K. Outcomes management in a prospective pay system. *Caring Magazine* 12(6):53, June 1993.

22. McGill, B., and others. COPD. *Case Management Newsletter* [HOMU Publication, No. X11] 1(12):1–2, Sept. 16, 1991.

23. Berwick, D. Seeking systemness. *Healthcare Forum Journal* 34(2):23, Mar.–Apr. 1992.

24. Wood, R., Bailey, N., and Tilkemeier, D. Managed care: the missing link in quality improvement. *Journal of Nursing Care Quality* 6(4):57, April 1992.

25. Argyris, C. Teaching smart people how to learn. *Harvard Business Review,* May–June 1991, pp. 99–109.

26. Berwick, D. Continuous quality improvement as an ideal in health care. *The New England Journal of Medicine* 320(1):55, Jan. 5, 1989.

27. Berwick, 1989, p. 56.

28. The effect on test ordering of informing physicians of the charges for outpatient diagnostic tests. *New England Journal of Medicine* 322(21), May 24, 1990.

29. The role of perceived price in physicians' demand for diagnostic tests. *Medical Care,* Feb. 1983, pp. 243–50.

30. Physician awareness of cost under prospective reimbursement systems. *Medical Care,* Mar. 1987, pp. 181–84.

31. Brownow, R., and others. The physicians who care plan. *Journal of the American Medical Association* 6(1):1–3, Winter 1991.

32. New England Medical Center Hospitals. *Building Blocks of Collaboration.* Boston: New England Medical Center Hospitals, 1987. (Unpublished video)

33. Zander, K. Physicians, CareMaps and collaboration. *The New Definition* 7(1):1–3, Winter 1992.

34. Leander, W. The fungible facility: constructing an ideal setting for restructuring. *PFCA Review,* Winter 1994, p. 11.

35. Leander.

Bibliography

Devereux, P. Does joint practice work? *Journal of Nursing Administration* 11(6):39–43, June 1981.

Devereux, P. Essential elements of nurse–physician collaboration: a changing relationship. *Journal of Nursing Administration* 11(6):35–38, June 1981.

Devereux, P. Nurse/physician collaboration: nursing practice considerations. *Journal of Nursing Administration* 11(8):37–39, Sept. 1981.

Goodwin, P. Nurse–physician collaborative practice. *Life Support Nursing* 86:9–16, May/June 1982.

Maucksch, I. Nurse–physician collaboration: a changing relationship. *Journal of Nursing Administration* 11(6):35–38, June 1981.

CHAPTER TWO

The Physician's New Agenda

John Kleinman, MD

In the past decade, the once-traditional cottage industry of health care has undergone dramatic and rapid transformation. Stable and conservative institutions and practices are now being challenged by the powerful forces of medical economics and federal, state, and local reform initiatives. Even without health care reform, rapid managed care organization growth, market consolidation, dwindling Medicare and Medicaid reimbursement, and the language of managed competition have forced many providers and organizations to question the future. New concepts of continuous quality improvement, practice guidelines, critical paths, and outcome management have been rapidly introduced to gain competitive advantages and, in some markets, to maintain probability of survival. In many places, the intensity of change has strained relationships and caused adversarial responses.

Increasingly, physicians, firmly rooted in the fierce self-autonomy of independent practices, are finding themselves disillusioned in a world that now favors local market forces reconfiguring the delivery of care. Physician self-autonomy, perhaps a consequence of education, training, and experience, has allowed development of both personal interests and vision and prevented physicians from uniting with a common philosophy. Thus, attempts to build a collective vision or collaborative practice style, essential to a meaningful response to reform initiatives, has often been viewed as a threat to physician practice autonomy. Lacking a common voice, physicians did not take a proactive role in the business of health care delivery but, rather, relinquished it to the payers of health care. As large managed care organizations began to flourish in competitive marketplaces, those involved in payment for medical services captured massive amounts of resource and utilization data from which were drawn conclusions with regard to the efficiency of competing hospitals, physicians, and other providers. Based on these data, payers in some areas of the country have already carved out areas of specialty care (such as cardiology, cardiovascular surgery, elective orthopedics, occupational medicine, and physical therapy) and sought to deliver volume to "efficient" providers. Physicians in like specialties practicing either solo, in groups, or at hospitals have begun to realize that although their practice style may be independent, they now are being measured as a group. Wasteful or highly variable practice styles will not enhance survival in the new competitive marketplace.

This chapter examines the new agenda or model for clinical quality improvement. It focuses on what the new agenda will mean for physicians and describes how to enlist their participation, leadership, and commitment to the changes demanded by the health care marketplace.

Evolution of the New Agenda

Many interesting, relatively consistent patterns characterize competitive markets as they evolve and mature. Young markets find that the initial focus of managed care organizations is on obtaining the deepest discount for unit of service from providers. The maintenance or increase of market share forces continual renegotiation of lower price per unit of service. As these markets mature, the number of units of service (in addition to the cost per unit of service) becomes a distinguishing factor. In turn, this triggers the rapid growth of administrative service and costs focused on preauthorization, precertification, concurrent utilization review, retrospective review, and denial of service. Managed care organizations doing the best job of "oversight" sell this feature in an attempt to grow market share. Providers and health care organizations in these markets typically find themselves participating in a bewildering array of what appear to be antagonistic or discordant activities to improve patient care. In response, providers begin to merge practices and consolidate organizations in an effort to create economies of scale and negotiating clout. This intensity and emotional charge provides fertile ground for three important events to occur:

1. The development and emergence of new concepts for clinical quality improvement
2. The need for and recognition of physician leadership committed to change
3. The collaborative redesign of the efficient use of health care resources

The continued interaction and transition of providers in these markets often results in a high level of integration and vertical alignment of the delivery system. Within these settings, integrated delivery systems develop. Because of organizational structure, these new entities have the potential to be better able to focus on systemic solutions for quality improvement and to measure efficiency as the cost required to improve the health status of the population of covered lives or community served. For these organizations, the use of guidelines, algorithms, and process design will be central to the new concept of health management. Where patient care had previously been event focused, institutionally based, and specialty driven, the new model will unfold across a continuum, from home care through primary community practices to fewer highly efficient, structured providers of specialty inpatient service and technology. Predictable patterns of resource consumption will require a collaborative process design integrating health care providers, materials management, and community resources with a system to study and reduce variation and improve outcome.

This new model will challenge what had once been known as fundamental laws and equations for provider and organizational success. Where the previous formula for success had been

$$\text{Success} = \text{Profit} = (\text{Price} \times \text{Volume}) - \text{Cost}$$

with clinical outcomes and quality as stated concerns, a profound shift to a new equation will occur. The new formula will be

$$\text{Success} = \text{Managing the Cost of Improved Outcome and Health Status}$$

with the focus of the delivery system on efficiency and achievement of desired outcomes. Under the old paradigm, admissions and ambulatory visits were the measurement standards for site of care. Payment issues focused on discount rate or fee-for-service equivalent. Success required volume, good payer mix, and cost and revenue management. The new paradigm will focus on which interventions (including preventive care), regardless of site of delivery, are most effective in achieving the desired outcome as well as what method is most efficient (least costly) to manage that outcome. Providers and organizations that understand and deliver health care using this new formula for success will be better positioned to manage risk and look for new areas to leverage within the equation to improve quality and to control cost.

This continuum of change has become so deeply rooted that it now is an unwritten expectation of providers to deliver cost-effective, high-quality care. To satisfy this mission with financial risk sharing requires physicians and their colleagues to build a collaborative effort through partnerships and alignment, affiliation, and integration. The fundamental requirement of these new relationships is to use the tools and techniques necessary to continuously study and improve patient care and to gather information that demonstrates the ability of the partnership to deliver high-quality, cost-effective outcomes.

All this, then, has led to the physician's new agenda: the collaborative redesign and delivery of high-quality patient care as measured by improved outcome and health status. The new agenda requires understanding the language of appropriate, efficient, and effective care and the use of new tools for case management and outcome measurement. It requires an understanding that high-quality patient care depends on more than achieving a clinical end point and that practice patterns are key to cost and quality. It also requires a broad understanding of the concepts for continuous quality improvement (CQI) and the importance of these concepts to organizational transformation.[1-4]

The Tools and Language of the New Agenda

In an article in the *New England Journal of Medicine*, Berwick captures the essence of the new agenda:

> Health care producers who commit themselves to improvement will invest energy in developing specific statements of purpose and algorithms for the clinical processes by which they intend to achieve those purposes . . . , such specifications are guidelines that are appropriate locally and are subject to ongoing assessment and revision.[5]

Inherent in this statement is the understanding that the delivery of high-quality patient care is remarkably complex and multidisciplined, with the methods and processes involved in reaching an outcome often differing remarkably at each decision point in the provision of care. Caregivers often do not recognize the complex sequences of practice style and support systems responsible for variation in resource use and outcome. What is required is the use of tools and concepts to help people and systems recognize opportunity and implement change.

Critical paths and case management provide clinical tools to integrate the tasks of physicians, health care professionals, support staff, and ancillary and community services to produce the expected (and best) intermediate- and long-term outcome. The design of these tools requires that three areas be addressed:

1. Is care appropriate?
2. Is care efficient?
3. Is care effective?

The underlying assumption is that appropriate care delivered in an efficient manner results in effective outcomes. By outward appearance, this assumption would resemble the linear equation

$$Appropriate + Efficient = Effective$$

But is this really a linear relationship? Further investigation of the definitions and descriptions that make up the equation will help answer this question and provide the basis for the further development of critical path and case management concepts.

Appropriateness of Care

Appropriateness of care is a reflection of the "practice" of medicine. It raises the question: Should it be done? Appropriateness is determined by answering treatment considerations such as which intervention, test, drug, or therapy to use based on consensus in the literature and the community standard. Because more often than not consensus does not exist and a testable model has not been developed, practice patterns are rooted in knowledge, training, intuition, preference, and resource availability. This then leads to measurable variation in practice patterns without demonstrable differences in outcome. This "paradox of appropriate care" as described by Wennberg[6] identifies the issue of differences in practice style as a variety of opinions concerning the need for and value of alternative treatments. Practice guidelines being developed by many sources are an attempt to reduce treatment uncertainty and variability. The American Medical Association (AMA) has defined practice guidelines as "recommendations for patient management which identify a particular management strategy or range of management strategies." For the most part, they are physician directed and decision focused, and fail to take into account process, system, and resource availability. Most often, they are designed by expert panels based on group consensus and their validity and effectiveness remain untested.[7-9] Perhaps a greater shortcoming of current practice guidelines (if strictly enforced) is that they do not provide a mechanism for innovation and evaluation through a feedback mechanism for redesign.[10-12]

No topic of discussion initiates a greater response or level of concern from physicians than that of appropriateness of guidelines. Physicians are intensely focused on achieving clinical end points and view them as the primary determinant of quality. The method or process involved in reaching that clinical end point often differs remarkably, even among physicians of the same specialty providing care for the same patient. Differences in practice style are often referred to as *the art of medicine*, and any attempt to design or plan clinical processes is viewed as a threat and labeled "cookbook medicine." At the center of this resistance and fear are two issues that must be resolved. First, physicians are committed to and, by nature, are competitive at being the best. The lack of clinical information systems with the ability to deliver reliable, anonymous feedback and their practice style has prevented physicians from understanding how that style compares with that of their peers. If a practice style is found to be "outside" the norm, how will that information be used? Second, if consensus on the development of a guideline can be reached, how will the guideline be used? Will it be used in a punitive fashion or as a flexible guide to study the process of patient care? Direct and sincere response to these questions with organizational commitment to learning, teaching, and improvement of clinical care is a fundamental necessity for physician buy-in.

Because appropriateness of care is a reflection of the practice of medicine, it affords the greatest opportunity for physician participation and leadership. The evaluation and improvement in practice styles requires a collaborative effort on the part of all those disciplines involved with that case type. Physicians are data driven, and the availability of accurate information that also takes into consideration patient variability or severity is necessary to begin the discussion. The definition of the *best practice* will require literature support, evaluation of any existing guidelines, and an understanding of resource availability or community standard. All efforts should be focused on using these collaborative achievements on medical rather than administrative management.

Efficiency of Care

Although there can and should be some overlap with appropriateness of care, efficiency of care requires that the ratio of the work done to the work required be optimal, that no more resources be applied than are required for an expected improvement to occur. Thus efficiency of care raises the question: How to do it? This focus of efficiency is on the process and associated costs of care. In the model described by Donabedian,[13] optimally effective care is the peak of a curve that describes useful additions to care versus benefits minus cost. (See figure 2-1.)

This model would require that the process management of care be understood and that the effects of care on the health status of patients and populations be understood and agreed on. Inefficient (poor-quality) care would occur whenever additional cost, evaluation, or treatment occurred that provided no measurable improvement in health.

Although from a clinical perspective this concept remains abstract, many concrete examples come to mind. For example:

- Multiple clinical laboratory tests repeated frequently without any demonstrable benefit
- Extensive health screening when none is required

Figure 2-1. Hypothetical Relations between Health Benefits and Cost of Care as Useful Additions Are Made to Care

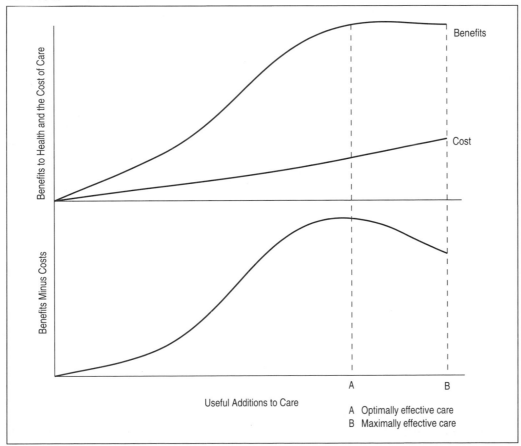

Reprinted, with permission, from Donabedian, A. The quality of care: how can it be assessed? *JAMA* 260:1743–48, 1988. Copyright, 1988, American Medical Association.

- Stacking of multiple technologies for imaging with X rays, CT scans, and magnetic resonance imaging (MRI)
- Substituting an expensive technology (MRI) for good clinical skills and evaluation

From an institutional and community perspective, efficiency of care requires an understanding of and method for improving complex support system interactions, multidisciplined sequential care delivery, and a method for extending care and prevention beyond institutional walls. Complex administrative systems and checks and balances that affect delivery must be understood and improved or eliminated. Achievement of improved efficiency requires the mapping and analysis of process flow. Mapping enhances the understanding of complex processes and the ability to analyze and improve efficiency and, therefore, outcome.

Critical paths are a prime example of process management tools applied to clinical care. They are process guidelines developed to reflect the optimal sequence of events, resources, and interventions required by all those involved in a defined case type.[14,15] In a more advanced form, critical paths define the relationship of sets of interventions to intermediate and expected outcomes along a time line.[16] Critical paths can be designed and used to study, analyze, and manage ambulatory diagnosis, inpatient care, urgent care, procedures, and community and health status improvement.

Physicians' perspective of efficiency is often one of system, bureaucracy, or support personnel interfering with their ability to rapidly achieve a clinical end point. They frequently forget that care is complex and multidisciplined and crosses departmental and institutional boundaries. Vital steps and information can be forgotten, lost, repeated, or done out of sequence. Physicians also have a very limited amount of information on the costs and uses of alternative treatment strategies. Improvement in efficiency requires that physicians understand process, cost, and interdependency. Once this level of understanding has been reached, physicians will be better equipped to engage in collaborative process redesign.

Effectiveness of Care

Perhaps the most complex question health care providers must consider concerns the effectiveness of care. The scope of effectiveness is patient focused: Did it work? Did we do the right thing? The interchangeable terminology of outcome measurement includes both objective and subjective measures that extend beyond a clinical end point. The use of this concept spans a broad arena from technology assessment to functional status, from technical skills to interpersonal skills, from patient motivation to community support.

The question of effectiveness needs to be divided into a minimum of two parts: the determinants of the effectiveness of care, and the tools used to measure effective care. The first part concerns the key elements critical to effectiveness. Donabedian lists these elements as:[17,18]

1. *Whether maximally effective or optimally effective care is sought:* Were all resources used, regardless of their proven ability to affect results, or were only useful treatments and innovations of proven marginal value brought to bear?
2. *Whether individual or social preference defines the optimum:* Should unlimited resources be used to benefit one individual, or should those same resources be more broadly applied to benefit the whole? Is the refusal of treatment, based on religious or personal beliefs, resulting in a preventable outcome or an untoward event?
3. *Whether effectiveness is determined by clinical skills, interpersonal skills, or amenities:* Is an astute clinician with poor interpersonal skills less effective than an average clinician with good interpersonal abilities? Through interpersonal skills, does the patient communicate enough information to make a sound clinical

judgment and does the clinician communicate adequate choices and treatment options? Does the environment in which care is delivered infer good or bad quality?

4. *Whether care is implemented by provider, patient, and family:* Has the provider given the patient/family an adequate understanding of the disease process or preventative measures? How is care to be assessed for noncompliant patients? Is the family available for or capable of implementing care?

5. *Whether the community contributes to care:* What is the impact of access to care or inadequate family, social, and community support systems on the short- and long-term effectiveness of care?

Donabedian describes these definitions of high-quality care as "successive circles surrounding a bull's-eye target."[19] (See figure 2-2.) The practitioners' and providers' knowledge, judgment, and skill remain the center or cornerstone and primary determinant of quality. Decisions regarding effectiveness or quality of care would therefore depend on assessing the performance of one, some, or all of these key elements.

The second question to be asked about effectiveness or outcome concerns the end points to be measured. Lohr describes the use of "the 5 Ds" (death, disease, disability, discomfort, and dissatisfaction) as the classical measurement standards.[20] With the exception of the "6th D" (dollars or cost of care), these five continue to form the basis for all measurement tools and systems currently used to evaluate the effectiveness of care. These end points span a range from objective to subjective measures of outcome:

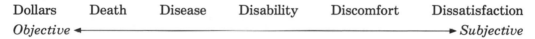

Dollars   Death   Disease   Disability   Discomfort   Dissatisfaction
Objective ◄————————————————————————————► *Subjective*

Figure 2-2.   Levels at Which Quality May Be Assessed

Care by practitioners and other providers:
• Technical performance
  Knowledge, judgment, and skill
• Interpersonal performance

Amenities

Care implemented by patient:
• Contribution of provider
• Contribution of patient and family

Care received by community:
• Access to care
• Performance of provider
• Performance of patient and family

Reprinted, with permission, from Donabedian, A. The quality of care: how can it be assessed? *JAMA* 260:1743–48, 1988. Copyright, 1988, American Medical Association.

Historically, the Health Care Financing Administration (HCFA), managed care organizations, and payers have used the more objective measures of mortality and morbidity to evaluate medical practice.[21] Traditional hospital quality assurance (QA) programs also have focused their efforts on mortality, readmissions, returns to surgery, and surgical and iatrogenic complications. Although these remain sentinel findings of what went wrong in patient care, the problems associated with definitions in data collection, severity adjustment interpretation including demographic and case-mix adjustment, and the inability to link medically pertinent causes to ambulatory care make it more difficult to draw conclusions about the quality or effectiveness of care.

New and evolving outcome measurement tools include measures of organ system function, disease-specific conditions, and functional evaluation and general measures of health status, including physical and mental health and patients' perspective of their functional capability and satisfaction levels.[22,23] The "technology of patient experience" would combine all these measurement tools in a comprehensive data pool that would include clinical and financial information as well as measurement of the patient's functioning and well-being through the use of health-status questionnaires and follow-up. This technology, which Ellwood refers to as *outcome management*, would "help patients, payers, and providers make rational medical care–related choices based on better insight into the effect of these choices on the patient's life."[24] However, application of these tools remains in its infancy; and questions related to adjustment of these subjective measures by severity and usefulness of these tools as a discriminating factor determining valuable differences between providers remain to be proven.[25]

The movement away from objective clinical end points to more subjective measures of outcome will certainly trouble the scientist inside every physician. The presentation and use of data that have not been statistically validated or scientifically proven remains a difficult feat. Nonetheless, this information will be used by payers to draw conclusions about better outcomes among competing providers. It will become increasingly important to demonstrate that value (cost) and outcome are directly related.

The Cycle of Outcome-Based Care

It should become increasingly apparent through the use of descriptive terms and definitions that the interrelationship of these concepts of care — appropriateness, efficiency, and effectiveness — has changed from the linear equation introduced in the last section to a new circular, unending form. (See figure 2-3.) The circular design captures the mental model required to understand the complex relationship of patient care to outcome. The appropriateness of care (Should it be done?) depends on the efficiency of care (Did it work?), which in turn may be profoundly affected by the effectiveness of care (How to do it?). The circular design also can be seen to represent Shewhart's PDCA cycle[26] in grand form: Plan (Should it be done?), Do (How to do it?), Check (Did it work?), Act (redesign of Should it be done? and How to do it?). No matter where in the cycle a provider or organization sets out to improve quality, the next step must be pursued in a never-ending fashion because all aspects become important determinants of quality.

Additional insight into interrelationships comes from the understanding that the tenets of CQI and the development of intermediate forward and feedback loops are central to the operational effectiveness of the design. (See figure 2-4.) *Appropriateness* now is defined by established practice guidelines. *Outcome* defines and is closely linked to appropriateness because it answers whether an intervention produced the desired outcome. The difference between the present practice of medicine and this model is that outcome management identifies variation in the success and failure of given interventions; this in turn is used to redesign or modify existing practice guidelines.

Figure 2-3. Cycle of Outcome-Based Care

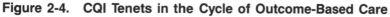

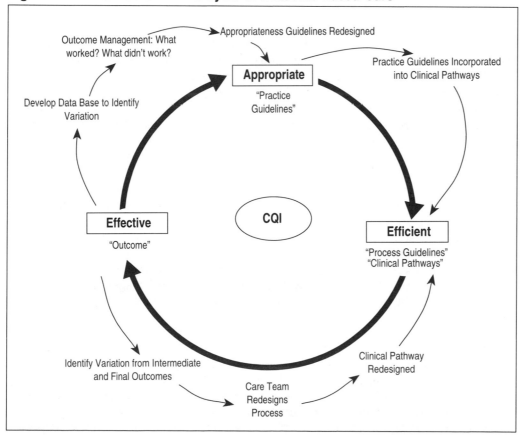

Figure 2-4. CQI Tenets in the Cycle of Outcome-Based Care

Application of these guidelines through clinical paths is then monitored for positive and negative variance from intermediate- and long-term outcome, and the principles of quality improvement are used as tools for process redesign.

The conceptual use of the cycle of outcome-based care pulls the initiatives of quality improvement into a synergistic and interdependent strategy. The individual and organizational approach now becomes: practice, process, outcome. It ties together what appear to be divergent disciplines into a sequential strategy for health care improvement. It allows providers to concentrate their interests where they are most comfortable, and later address more difficult tasks. For example, physicians now are aware that there is variation in medical practice yet fear the use of guidelines, which they describe as "cookbook medicine." If the initial interest and focus is on the process or efficiency of care, collaborative involvement and consensus building will lead to questioning both appropriateness and the relationship of appropriateness and process to outcome.

Collaboration with Physician Colleagues

As mentioned previously, one of the challenges faced in the current health care environment is that of confronting physician fears related to the erosion or perceived loss of clinical autonomy, the preservation of self-interest, and the reality of health care reform. It is difficult for many physicians to take an organizational perspective on the delivery of health care because of their education, training, and intense patient–problem focus. The reality of reform is that it requires physicians to have a stake in the successes of organizations to which they relate. Thus understanding physicians' fears and overcoming their resistance to working collaboratively is a crucial first step on the road to reform.

As discussed by Zander, collaboration "entails an unspoken acknowledgment of interdependence and demonstrated mutual respect."[27] Thus one of the early tasks in involving a group of physicians in a session designed to introduce outcome-based care may be to discuss the issues of respect and interdependence as they relate to patient care. Another task is to agree on which area of the cycle to study first. Because these diagnoses require a multidisciplinary approach, critical path development is the logical first step. Critical paths also facilitate the incorporation of standing orders, algorithms, or guidelines into a patient care plan.

Physician involvement in critical path development should be initiated with program or specialty focus. Physician participation in centers of excellence or product lines such as obstetrics, orthopedics, rehabilitation, or oncology provide an excellent opportunity for areas to initiate the effort. Within these areas, one or more high-volume, high-cost, or highly variable diagnoses or case types should be selected. The usual association of case management and case managers with product lines will facilitate startup. Session activities should be implemented in a positive manner with improvement of quality as the declared goal. The environment of the session should be educational and safe without the use of physician identifiers or hidden agendas. If and when arguments arise, the group should be reminded that its collaborative purpose is patient care centered.

Activities might be structured in the following sequence:

1. Because physicians are data driven and will be interested in *accurate* information demonstrating differences in length of stay, resource use, and variability of practice patterns, one or more willing physicians should be enlisted to present the data and champion the effort.
2. Chart audit information (10 to 20 charts) on trends, best practice, and expected standards met should be provided. The physicians should be asked to identify

desired outcomes, case type boundaries, and the language or areas for variation to be studied.

3. Interested physicians should be involved in the collaborative team designing the draft model and should present it to their colleagues for input and modification.
4. The critical path and study variance should be instituted allowing the design group to modify and improve the plan.
5. The value of the critical path should be reinforced by comparing data in a user-friendly fashion showing enhancements in care that have resulted.

In summary, four elements are essential for the development of successful critical path models. These are:

1. Critical paths should be developed through a collaborative process with clinicians and all others involved in the patient care type. The path should represent a consensus of best practice as determined by prevailing practice and expected or preferred practice patterns. Intermediate-term and final or long-term outcome events should be defined by the group.
2. Even though critical paths should not represent inflexible templates, a method of measuring and attributing variance from pathway task and outcome should be included. Most variance designs attribute both positive and negative variance to four major categories: system, patient, practitioner, and community (or external system).
3. The Shewhart PDCA cycle should be used to create a feedback loop for case management reassessment and redesign on a continual basis. Using these building blocks, a continuum of tasks, interventions, and outcomes can be developed, evaluated, and modified in a dynamic fashion to define and coordinate the processes of patient care.
4. These concepts should be incorporated into the culture of the organization and care of patients. Allocation of resources, creation of incentives, and development of skills are requirements for success that must be committed forever for outcome-based care to become the practice style for all caregivers.

Allocation of resources: Organizational commitment to critical path development, consensus building of appropriateness criteria, and outcome study requires the investment of time, money, and dedicated personnel. The actual cost to the organization may not change substantially considering present expenditures on quality assurance, case management, and information services. Redirecting existing resources to the study of appropriate, efficient, and effective care provides the framework for quality improvement. These new QA activities fulfill the evolving movement toward collaborative practice supported by the Joint Commission on Accreditation of Healthcare Organizations (JCAHO). In addition, pulling together the two information system databases of finance and clinical information will aid in the movement toward clinical cost-effectiveness by producing performance comparisons.

Creation of incentives: The codependency of health care delivery cannot be forgotten. Hospitals and organizations require physician participation in the treatment and care of patients at the same time that physicians require stable and financially sound institutions to maintain and improve the skills of other caregivers and the technology required for them to practice. Because critical paths and appropriateness and effectiveness assessments are intended to improve efficiency of care and aid in the determination of ineffective diagnostic or treatment methods, they should assist in reducing unnecessary costs and services. In markets where capitation and risk sharing are the rule, the incentives are obvious. In other markets where health care financing, not-for-profit status, and inurement issues prohibit gain sharing, commitment should be made to reinvest savings in program development, personnel, and appropriate technology and equipment purchase.

In addition, physicians should recognize many advantages of critical paths that extend beyond their value as case management tools. Critical paths allow all caregivers to focus their expertise on a given case type and thus improve patient care. They become powerful tools in identifying support system issues such as timeliness, accurateness, information transfer, capital equipment needs, and other reliability problems related to service enhancement. Additionally, collaboration leads to empowerment and greater job satisfaction for all caregivers. Critical paths can enhance the educational value and interest in any given case type as a training tool for interns, residents, and other health care professionals. If properly designed, they can reduce the number of questions and phone calls directed to physicians. Finally, they provide an opportunity for physicians to participate in the building of a shared vision by developing a program of excellence, reducing variation in practice style, encouraging the study and advancement of improved outcomes, and improving the health of a community by customizing processes that best meet population needs.

Development of skills: Organizational commitment to learning may be a key feature that differentiates providers in the future competitive market.[28-30] This can be broadly divided into two areas: (1) development of knowledge and skills that currently do not exist within the organization, and (2) development of the knowledge to "lead" (or the interpersonal skills required of leadership development). An educational investment should be made to learn and teach the principles of quality improvement, case management, critical path design, guideline development, and outcome research. At the same time, investment also should be made to develop the interpersonal skills and effectiveness of leaders, including physicians. Leadership skills should focus on designing and teaching learning processes to steward organizational resources. Efforts should be made to promote creative thinking and problem solving throughout the organization.

Berwick summarized the following changes to improve appropriateness that also apply to the changes necessary to deliver outcome-based care. These are:

- Support the collection of data on outcomes of care and utilization of procedures and report those data, stratified by individual physician and institution, in a setting that permits trusting and respectful comparison and discussion without the threat of external reprisal or maneuvers of control. Small amounts of "risk adjustment" or "severity adjustment" may make such data more credible to physicians, although most such adjustment will not change the basic qualitative findings. Encourage the clinicians to talk openly about the findings, and to use the data to guide further experiments.
- With or without comparative data (but best of all with it), encourage clinicians to visit each other. . . . One of the best ways for doctors to understand variation in practice is to see each other's work firsthand.
- Consider local "appropriateness" reviews by clinicians among themselves. . . . Focus reviews more on the possible systemic generators of inappropriateness than upon individual people.
- Discover and implement simple ways to reduce variation and increase appropriateness by technical and administrative changes that do not require exhortation or behavior change. For example, if physicians can agree that it is rarely appropriate to order both a blood urea nitrogen and a serum creatinine to assess renal function, the most effective way to change ordering patterns is to remove the less preferred test as a standard "check-off" item on the preprinted laboratory ordering form.
- Develop forms of communication between specialists and primary care-givers that permit each to teach the other about choices of tests and treatments. The best such teaching will occur "on the spot," when a specific radiologist suggests

to a referring internist, that only one view was needed even though two were ordered, or when a specific pediatrician asks a dermatologist about a treatment strategy so that the pediatrician can implement it without a referral next time.

- When economic incentives are judged to play a major role in inappropriate care [which Berwick believes to be less common than is often assumed], try, as a professional and corporate community, to manipulate the incentives in a favorable direction. This will become more and more possible—indeed, more and more necessary—in a "managed care" or "single payer" environment, in which waste in one area is a loss to all.
- Enlist the patient directly in decisions about "appropriateness." Somewhat against the common wisdom, recent research is beginning to suggest that direct patient involvement in diagnostic and therapeutic decisions may lead to more parsimonious and more appropriate decisions than when the patient remains uninvolved in such choices.
- Assure rapid notice and use of sound, new clinical investigations, especially randomized controlled trials. Research shows lag times of ten years or more between the appearance of a definitive clinical study and the reflection of that study in common practice. Doctors are understandably overwhelmed by the deluge of research facts that pour out of their journals, and a helpful clinical culture may need a way to say to all, "Notice this, and let's put it to use now."[31]

A Collaborative Example: The Minnesota Clinical Comparison and Assessment Project

The Minnesota Clinical Comparison and Assessment Project (MCCAP) is the outgrowth of a 1988 effort by Minnesota hospitals to evaluate and recommend the purchase of a common severity system measurement tool.[32-34] The results of that study, conducted by a local not-for-profit research foundation called the Health Education and Research Foundation (HERF), found that all the severity systems studied had relative value, but because of their "closed-design" format, providers had difficulty trusting results. No single severity measurement tool appeared to be superior. Thus a consensus developed that hospitals should postpone purchase and, instead, establish a collaborative effort to collect and compare clinical information and outcomes following development of appropriateness, clinical efficiency, and effectiveness guidelines on selected case types.

This unrivaled effort brought together the following organized health care providers: Hennepin County Medical Society, Ramsey County Medical Society, Minnesota Medical Association, University of Minnesota School of Public Health, with the Minnesota Hospital Association, Council of Hospital Corporations, and 53 acute care hospitals representing 60 percent of the licensed beds in the state. This consortium agreed to fund and participate in the development and evaluation of guidelines and clinical practice assessment.

The project's objective was to determine whether clinical data collection systems with feedback to clinicians could be developed, comparing their practice with best practice to improve clinical behavior. MCCAP was built on the following six assumptions:[35]

1. Health care assessment and improvement requires high-technology, communitywide, multiprofessional approaches that involve not only clinicians but also organized medicine, nursing, and health care institutions and organizations.
2. Clinicians will use information to modify their behavior and medical practice to improve the quality of care delivered, if routine and systematic clinical information systems and performance review mechanisms are developed that are clinically credible and meaningful to them.

3. Clinical services will be evaluated most effectively if clinicians are involved in all aspects of the development and operation of the system.
4. Comparison with predetermined, specified guidelines or parameters is essential for evaluating clinical practice and offering improvement opportunities.
5. Ongoing and repeated medical education programs, coupled with individual feedback of clinical performance data by respected clinical leaders, can be effective in changing clinical behavior and potentially improving clinical effectiveness and efficiency.
6. Clinical behavior will be influenced most effectively through the feedback of clinically useful information that stresses professional and collegial incentives rather than sanctions, and continuous practice improvement rather than programs to "catch the bad guys."

Through a collaborative effort, HERF developed a model for quality of care evaluation and improvement (figure 2-5) and agreed on the initial study of elective cholecystectomy (both open and laparoscopic), cesarean section, uncomplicated

Figure 2-5. MCCAP Model for Quality of Care Evaluation and Improvement

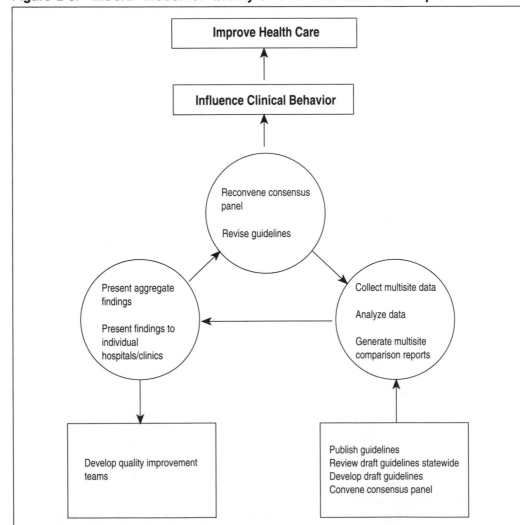

myocardial infarction, and total hip replacement. Throughout 1001, HERF convened consensus panels to develop guidelines that "were not represented as standards of care, but rather the authors' and reviewers' best statement at a certain time about the appropriate and effective treatment for certain clinical conditions."[36]

The panels were formed for each of the study conditions and consisted of one or more prominent local clinical leaders representing the specialty area of guideline development, primary care and referral physicians, nurses, and quality management staff from community hospitals and tertiary care institutions. Physician participation in local guideline development and endorsement also was critical in lending authority to the program and providing local information advisors and contacts for practicing clinicians to link the project with their institution. By the end of 1991, guidelines were approved and published for elective cholecystectomy, total hip replacement, cesarean birth, pediatric asthma, and uncomplicated myocardial infarction.

The panels found no existing guidelines that met their needs exactly. Little if any literature was found to support existing guidelines as they related to expected outcomes. None contained methods to severity-adjust or risk-adjust for comorbidity. The panels also rejected an algorithm format for the guidelines because of their inability to capture the complexity of patient care for the case types selected. Guideline development consisted of reviewing and synthesizing information obtained from literature searches and incorporating findings based on consensus within the panels.

Using the guideline for elective cholecystectomy as an example, all guidelines were developed using a similar format:

- Case type definition
- Background
- Indications for procedures (including appropriate diagnostic findings)
- Treatment guidelines (preoperative, perioperative, interoperative, and postoperative)
- Recovery guidelines (including discharge education, discharge planning, outcome criteria at discharge)

Expected intervention outcomes and patient comorbidity characteristics (severity measures) that might modify and affect treatment and procedures outcomes also were defined. In addition, preadmission health status questionnaires, six-month follow-up questionnaires, and chart abstraction tools were reviewed. The entire format developed was then sent to the appropriate departments at participating hospitals for medical staff and support staff review and revision. Comments were incorporated into the revision of the final document and published. Formal guidelines also carried a disclaimer stating that they did not include all proper methods of care or exclude other acceptable methods of care reasonably directed at obtaining the same results.

From project inception it was understood that all providers would not necessarily follow guideline recommendations until evidence demonstrated a causal relationship between appropriateness, treatment, and outcome. This presented MCCAP with the unique opportunity to study the relationship of practice variation to outcome. Collected data comparing institutional practice patterns with best practice as defined by the guideline would be analyzed and brought back to participating institutions in anonymous fashion. The analysis also compared site-specific adherence to guideline and outcome results with the performance of all other participating institutions. By the end of 1992, patient enrollment and most postdischarge outcome information had been collected on 3,500 elective cholecystectomy, 2,700 cesarean birth, and 2,500 total hip replacement patients. Beginning in 1993, HERF support staff scheduled on-site educational sessions with representatives at each institution to review results from the cholecystectomy and cesarean section studies. Typically, these sessions involved multidisciplinary teams including nurses and quality management staff in addition to physicians. Where available, case managers, medical directors, and department chairs also were invited. Additionally, each institution was given computer discs containing the medical record and provider information specific to that hospital. It is the expectation of the project that study findings will be incorporated into clinical quality improvement activities and be used as a springboard to modify clinical behavior.

Although MCCAP appears to be a monumental undertaking that may have limited application beyond study participants, it contains valuable lessons and implications for collaborative practice. For example:

- Although completed guidelines (or critical paths) may closely resemble nationally available guidelines, the importance of local involvement and approval with multidisciplinary teams cannot be overemphasized. Physicians remain very concerned about what is going to be measured and what will be done with the results. Thus they must be involved at the local level in development, implementation, and review. Furthermore, a method of updating and revising appropriate indications and treatment based on outcome findings, local resource availability, new research findings, and practice-style change (for example, open to laparoscopic cholecystectomy) needs to be understood and applied.
- Initial selection should focus on high-volume, high-variability diagnoses or treatments. The panels found that the process of appropriateness and efficiency design was easier for procedures (total hip replacement) and more difficult for conditions (pediatric asthma).
- Optional adherence to recommend guidelines and process is necessary for implementation. Credible study and feedback of variation is necessary to modify behavior and medical practice toward a more uniform or preferred practice pattern. Physicians are more willing to change practice behavior when they understand the relationship of treatment to outcome.
- The amount of time, effort, and expense necessary to complete outcome evaluations is often underestimated. Projects require the commitment of time, resources, and personnel and must be budgeted as an expense. In addition, the composition and leadership of multidisciplinary teams is a critical factor contributing to the project's continuation and success. Excluding time donated by expert panels and institutional resources donated to implement and collect patient data, the MCCAP cost per guideline was $40,000. Program costs of data collection, verification, analysis, and follow-up approximated $50 per patient.[37] Local initiatives combining payer claims information, medical record review, and standard patient-generated outcome measures may be less expensive.
- Whether or not efforts directed at clinical quality improvement can influence clinical decision making and patient care depends on the level of organizational integration. Involvement in case management activities and critical path design and implementation may be a key finding of successful organizations for two reasons: First, the involvement of different departments, disciplines, and physicians in a given case type requires agreement of a forum to change a multidisciplined process; and, second, case management and critical paths are evidence that administration, departments, caregivers, and physicians support a collaborative effort of clinical quality improvement.

The study and linkage of outcome to appropriateness and processes of patient care, as suggested by the cycle of outcome-based care, is a powerful tool for understanding and improving patient care and expectations. The following examples illustrate this point.[38,39]

- At one hospital, patients took significantly longer to return to activities of daily living after both open and laparoscopic cholecystectomy. A review of illness severity, complications, and discharge status did not find that the delay in return to normal activities could be attributed to clinical factors. Armed with this information, the hospital's team effort was directed toward revising discharge planning and patient education and reviewing the sick leave policies for certain large employers.

- Another hospital was found to have significantly shorter length of stay following cholecystectomy than other hospitals in the study. Postdischarge questionnaires for that hospital found a higher proportion of patients feeling they were released prematurely. Study evaluation of complications and postdischarge functional status found no difference among other hospitals. Because no clinical reason for prolonging patient stay could be found, the hospital focused efforts on improving patient expectations. Discharge planning and education was redesigned so that patients better understood recovery time and length of hospitalization required for cholecystectomy.

- MCCAP perioperative guidelines did not recommend the universal use of prophylactic antibiotics but, rather, defined a high-risk subset that included the following patient characteristics: age greater than 65 years, diabetes mellitus, obstructive jaundice or common duct stones, prosthetic devices or cardiac valvular disease, and immunologic suppression. Despite panel-developed guideline recommendation, many surgeons initially rejected the selective use of prophylactic antibiotics. However, the study found that the infection rate in patients where no antibiotics were used appropriately was no different from that of the group that was given antibiotics without meeting appropriateness criteria. This provided all hospitals the information necessary to design and support the study of appropriate prophylactic antibiotic use in this population.

- The MCCAP study of cesarean section has raised a very important question. Conventional utilization review and payer concern regarding cesarean section is directed at the absolute rate of cesarean section versus normal delivery. The operating assumption follows that low cesarean section rates are the benchmark for a high level of appropriate practice style. For the 20 hospitals with statistically significant numbers of patients participating in the MCCAP study, the rate of C-section varied from 6 to 29 percent of total births. One hospital had a rate of 6 percent with only 58 percent of C-sections meeting appropriateness guidelines, whereas another had a rate of 16 percent with 80 percent meeting appropriateness definitions. Obviously, patient mix and other characteristics are contributing to this variation. A more valuable approach may be to spend more energy on high levels of adherence to appropriateness criteria and less time on the absolute C-section rate.

These examples are only a small sample of the wealth of information flowing from MCCAP results. Whether MCCAP will make a difference in changing practice patterns and improving patient outcome is highly dependent on the collaborative efforts of study participants at a local level. This question remains to be answered.

Conclusion

The ability to demonstrate and document the delivery of improved outcome and health status using collaborative tools for the redesign of health care delivery is the physician's new agenda. Knowing the concepts of the cycle of outcome-base care, the relationship of appropriateness and process (efficiency) to outcome (effectiveness) is the cornerstone of collaborative redesign. Concentration on only one aspect of the cycle, either appropriateness or process alone, cannot be counted on to improve the quality and value of patient care. It is necessary to educate physicians and all caregivers about these relationships and to create a learning culture comfortable with change. The tools that can be used to embed this change into the delivery process are critical paths and case management. Further understanding of the causes of variation from intermediate- and long-term outcome quantifies the value of more uniform practice styles, generates documentation to eliminate barriers to effective delivery, and provides a method of understanding and improving patient preferences and expectations.

Where will outcome-based care lead? The answer is not yet known; for the first time the health care industry is standing at the threshold of a new science that should allow providers to define, measure, and improve the health of the community they serve.

References

1. Berwick, D. M. Continuous improvement as an ideal in health care. *New England Journal of Medicine* 320(1):53–56, Jan. 5, 1989.

2. Laffel, G., and Blumenthal, D. The case for using industrial quality management science in health care organizations. *Journal of the American Medical Association* 262(20):2869–73, Nov. 24, 1989.

3. Berwick, D. M. Controlling variation in health care: a consultation from Walter Shewhart. *Medical Care* 29(12):1212–25, Dec. 1991.

4. Blumenthal, D. Total quality management and physicians' clinical decisions. *Journal of the American Medical Association* 269(12):2775–78, June 2, 1993.

5. Berwick, Continuous improvement as an ideal in health care.

6. Wennberg, J. E. The paradox of appropriate care. *Journal of the American Medical Association* 258(18):2568–69, Nov. 13, 1987.

7. Kane, R. L., and Lurie, N. Appropriate effectiveness: a tale of carts and horses. *Quality Review Bulletin* 10(10):322–26, Oct. 1992.

8. Eisenberg, J. M., and Foster, N. E. Using clinical guidelines: impact on public policy, clinical policy and individual care decisions. In: *Bridging the Gap Between Theory and Practice: Exploring Practice Guidelines.* Chicago: American Hospital Association, Hospital Research and Education Trust, 1993.

9. Phelps, L. E. The methodologic foundation of studies of the appropriateness of medical care. *New England Journal of Medicine* 329(17):1241–44, Oct. 21, 1993.

10. Phelps.

11. Kassirer, J. P. The quality of care and the quality of measuring it. *New England Journal of Medicine* 329(17):1263–64, Oct. 21, 1993.

12. Hirshfeld, E. B. Should practice parameters be the standard of care in malpractice litigation? *Journal of the American Medical Association* 266(20):2886–91, Nov. 27, 1991.

13. Donabedian, A. The quality of care: how can it be assessed? *Journal of the American Medical Association* 260(12):1743–48, Sept. 1988.

14. Coffey, R. J., Richards, J. S., Remmert, C. S., LeRoy, S. S., Shoville, R. R., and Baldwin, P. J. An introduction to critical paths. *Quality Management in Health Care* 1(1):45–54, Fall 1992.

15. Zander, K. Critical pathways. In: *Total Quality Management: The Health Care Pioneers.* Chicago: American Hospital Publishing, 1992.

16. Zander.

17. Donabedian.

18. Donabedian, A. Quality and cost: choices and responsibilities. *Journal of Occupational Medicine* 32(12):1167–72, Dec. 1990.

19. Donabedian, The quality of care.

20. Lohr, K. N. Outcome measurement: concepts and questions. *Inquiry* 25(1):37–50, Spring 1988.

21. Roper, W. L., Winkenwerder, W., Hackbarth, G. M., and Krakaver, H. Effectiveness in healthcare: an initiative to evaluate and improve medical practice. *New England Journal of Medicine* 319(18):1197–1202, Nov. 3, 1988.

22. Nelson, E. C., and Berwick, D. M. The measurement of health status in clinical practice. *Medical Care* [supplement] 27(3):77–90, Mar. 1989.

23. Tarlov, A. R., Ware, J. E., Greenfield, S., Nelson, E. C., Perrin, E., and Zubkoff, M. The Medical Out-comes Study: an application of methods for monitoring the results of medical care. *Journal of the American Medical Association* 262(7):925-30, Aug. 1989.

24. Ellwood, P. M. Shattuck Lecture—outcomes management: a technology of patient experience. *New England Journal of Medicine* 318(23):1549-56, June 1988.

25. Lohr.

26. Walton, M. *The Deming Management Method.* New York City: Putnam, 1986.

27. Zander, K. Physicians, CareMaps, and collaboration. *The New Definition* 7(1):1-3, 1992.

28. Drucker, P. F. The coming of the new organization. *Harvard Business Review* 66(1):45-53, Jan.-Feb., 1988.

29. Senge, P. M. The leaders new work: building learning organizations. *Sloan Management Review* 32(1):7-23, Fall 1990.

30. Senge, P. M. Transforming the practice of management. *Human Resource Development Quarterly* 4(1):5-37, Spring 1993.

31. Berwick, D. M. Improving the appropriateness of care. *Quality Connection* 3(1):1-6, Winter 1994.

32. Borbas, C., McLaughlin, D. B., and Schultz, A. The Minnesota Clinical Comparison and Assessment Program: bridging the gap between clinical practice guidelines and patient care. In: *Bridging the Gap Between Theory and Practice: Exploring Practice Guidelines.* Chicago: American Hospital Association, Hospital Research and Education Trust, 1993.

33. Borbas, C., Stump, M. A., Dedeker, K., Lurie, N., McLaughlin, D., and Schultz, A. The Minnesota Clinical Comparison and Assessment Program. *Quality Review Bulletin* 16(2):87-92, Feb. 1990.

34. Norling, R. A., McLaughlin, D. B., Schultz, A., and Borbas, C. The Minnesota Clinical Comparison and Assessment Program: a resource for clinical quality improvement programs. *The Quality Letter* 5(5):14-17, June 1993.

35. Borbas, Stump, Dedeker, Lurie, McLaughlin, and Schultz.

36. Borbas, McLaughlin, and Schultz.

37. Borbas, McLaughlin, and Schultz.

38. Borbas, McLaughlin, and Schultz.

39. Norling and others.

esign

lth care professional and trade literature has exploded with arti-
y possible type of critical path/CareMap tool, care management,
nt program. To outside observers or agencies considering launch-
components of collaborative care, the diversity of programs can
erhaps off-putting. However, to the experienced collaborative care
ty is understandable and usually praiseworthy because it offers collaborative care models that can be customized to meet specific organization needs.
The important fact is that all collaborative care programs are founded on the same
basic clinical and management principles.

This chapter discusses the four criteria that are necessary to turn a collaborative
care concept into a realistic, workable program. It also describes the essential components of a collaborative care program infrastructure and offers examples of successful
programs in different health care organization structures.

Integration of Collaborative Care Models

Models are composed of concepts, images, and prescriptions for behavior. They become
real when they are integrated into the fabric of behavior they are designed to affect.
Thus, as in architecture, form must fit the expected function. For a collaborative care
model or program to become more than an ideal concept, the following four criteria
must be met: (1) Models must have annual goals that can be evaluated regularly; (2)
Goals must be doable within the region and sociopolitical environment; (3) A direct
relationship must exist between the goals and the processes and structures designed
to achieve them; and (4) People working in the model must be given the authority
and new-skill education to fulfill their responsibilities.

Determine Goals

Models must have annual goals that can be evaluated regularly. It is important to
determine goals for the overall program as well as for specific cases and to evaluate
them both quantitatively (for example, by how many days can hospital length of stay
be reduced?) and qualitatively (for example, how much readmission is acceptable overall

59

and for this case type?). (Evaluation methods are discussed in detail in chapter 9.) Additionally, goals must be made responsive to external factors and regulations. One straightforward approach to determining goals is to list all such factors and regulations and assess how the organization approaches them at each level of operation. For example, if a community hospital wants to ensure closer allegiance with its physicians and improve its competitive advantage in the region, it may feel that forming a physician–hospital organization (PHO) is the only commitment it needs to make to achieve that goal. However, if the hospital also wants its physician–hospital alliance to include an effort to firm up current clinical programs and begin new ones, it should incorporate CareMap tools and perhaps case management in its change strategy.

Another approach to determining goals is to rank-order the possible effects of the CareMap tools and case management methods underlying collaborative care to determine which ones best address the stresses and problems facing the organization. Examples of such effects include:

- Accommodating managed care contracts
- Decreasing fragmentation/increasing access of services
- Improving patient/family satisfaction
- Operationalizing continuous quality improvement (CQI) at the patient care level
- Enhancing collaboration among disciplines
- Providing database (through variance) for CQI
- Linking actual costs to actual care given
- Decreasing length of stay (LOS) where appropriate
- Improving patient/family participation and education
- Conducting action research
- Restructuring accountability models
- Conforming to the most recent requirements of the Joint Commission on Accreditation of Healthcare Organizations (JCAHO)
- Streamlining documentation
- Decreasing readmission
- Developing realistic outcomes management approach
- Modeling resource, staffing, materials management needs
- Preparing for computerization of medical records
- Lessening risk of malpractice

For example, the home care agency that can still be paid on a per visit basis will not want to decrease visits until reimbursement methods change, but may want to use CareMap tools and case management to streamline documentation and standardize outcomes. Likewise, the university medical center striving to conduct clinical research as well as promote its world-famous vascular surgery may choose CareMap tools and case management as a way to further solidify its academic and global position.

Rank-ordering also helps the organization prioritize which clinical area or case type to focus on first. For example, the hospital that ranks high on its list the goal of decreasing LOS and resource use where appropriate and nonconflictual with the desirable patient and family outcomes may choose to focus on case types such as fractured hip, laryngectomy, and diabetes, each for different reasons and with different strategies. The goal would then need to be further explicated as to which case types are most financially problematic and for what reasons. For instance, fractured hip patients may have a long LOS that is preventable, whereas laryngectomy patients (a catastrophic condition) will have a long LOS and heavy resource use that are not very amenable to modification. A CareMap tool may be sufficient for coordinating the care of fractured hip patients, whereas laryngectomy patients may need a case manager to coordinate acute and home services. (A CareMap tool might be used with the latter case type as well, but more for coordination than potential cost savings.) On the other hand, the hospital may choose to focus on diabetes because of high readmission rates and poor patient satisfaction scores.

Ensure Attainability of Goals

Goals must be doable within the region and sociopolitical environment. Sometimes health care organizations are so eager to reach certain collaborative care goals that they ignore or underestimate their external environment. For example, the goal of establishing outcomes management may be new to departments and disciplines that do not have access to conferences about clinical outcomes offered outside the institution. In some cases, collaborative care may not be perceived as a desirable or acceptable philosophy, especially if staff associate it with a loss of power. Additionally, the region in which an organization is located can have a tremendous influence on the choice of collaborative care goals. For example, some overall program goals such as increasing access to services may be very difficult in regions of the country that have problems attracting physical therapists or other specialists. Likewise, the goal of improving patient/family participation and education will be a challenge in regions where illiteracy and/or poverty is common.

No goals are totally unachievable; they merely need to be modified so that people in the organization can, wherever possible, feel successful as they participate in the process of collaboration. If the goals are grounded in *real* knowledge of the world outside the organization, good design will flow from them.

Design Goals Around Processes

A direct relationship must exist between the goals and the processes and structures designed to achieve them. Process, structure, and outcome are the well-accepted components of any system. *Process* is the way in which the underlying structures create the outcomes. In fact, collaborative care itself is a process built on some old and new structures to achieve specific clinical and financial goals.

Using Collaborative Care to Enhance CQI

On a large scale, the goal of using collaborative care to enhance CQI is quite prevalent. To do justice to structure, process, and outcome, one community teaching institution designed a flowchart to show the connections between CareMap tools and variance data, and CQI. (See figure 3-1.) In this specific institution, the flowchart established the priority that CQI is a process that in turn enhances collaborative care, and the two processes combined give everyone greater ability to produce desirable outcomes.

Toward the same end, another institution further defined three structures necessary for successful implementation. These were:

1. *Teams:* In hospitals, these are groups of health care professionals organized around case types (products).
2. *Systems:* These are blueprints designed to determine how to build and manage the product (case type). The teams develop clinical care guidelines (similar to the CareMap tools) to facilitate progression within a case type from admission to discharge.
3. *Variance management:* This is done to recognize and adjust for deviations from the norm. The data are then used to improve the outcome or product.

Lowering Costs by Lowering Resource Consumption

If lowering costs by lowering resource consumption is one of the key goals of collaborative care, one of the underlying structures must be financial information about cost

Karen Zander

Figure 3-1. Flowchart: From CQI to Ownership by Operations

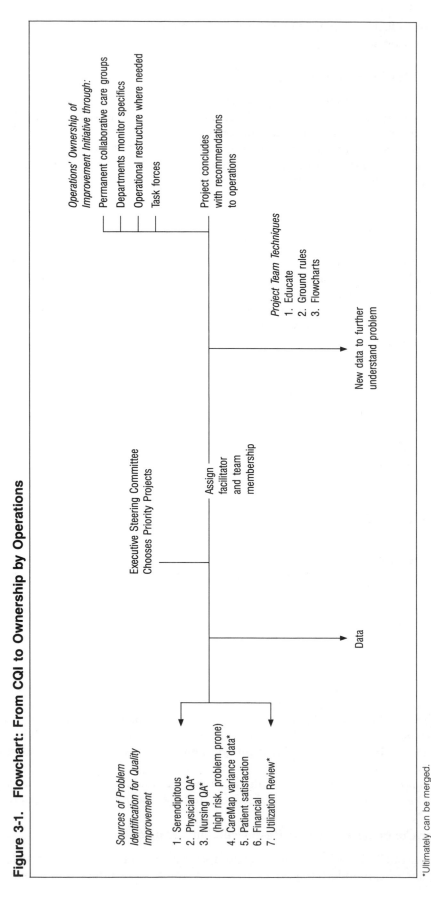

*Ultimately can be merged.
Reprinted, with permission, from The Center for Case Management, South Natick, MA.*

62

per case. If this information is not available, it will have to be constructed from pieces of information. The formula for construction should be a combination of fixed and variable costs. For example, total cost per case would include resources ordered by physicians as well as the overhead cost to a patient in that case type for services rendered by nursing and other "nonchargeable" departments.

Sharon Henry, product line manager of the Cardiac Centers, Mercy and Unity Hospitals in Minneapolis, suggests that certain data be added to cost per case to decide which case types to manage. These data include:[1]

- Case type volumes
- Severity categories
- LOS
- Variation spread in LOS
- Practice variations
- Number of outliers
- Readmission rates
- Disposition (after hospital)
- Comorbid condition
- Benchmarks

She suggests that further case type–specific data be collected by reviewing:

- Health Care Financing Administration (HCFA) statistics
- Severity-adjusted LOS
- Local practice
- Any available outcome information
- Operating room (OR) costs
- Segments of the clinical course
- Perfusion, anesthesia, and prosthesis costs
- Nursing care costs
- Physician leadership and preferences

Calculating the comprehensive cost per case will be an important goal for all health care organizations in the next few years. Putting the data from above together with home care, equipment, and outpatient care will be imperative in a largely financially capitated industry.

Provide New-Skill Education

People working in the model must be given the authority and new-skill education to fulfill their responsibilities. Several distinct groups of people need the authority and education to work in the collaborative care model and produce its expected overall outcomes. Among these groups are the executive steering committee and the project manager (discussed in the next section), and the physicians (discussed in chapter 2).

However, the group that needs to understand collaborative care the most but which—almost without exception—receives the least education and attention consists of middle managers and department heads. Traditionally, their introduction to this major organizational change is limited to their attendance at an information session. The integration of processes is significantly different from the management of departments, and it should not be assumed that this group will automatically decipher how to support this change without appropriate education.

Following are some suggestions for the education of the manager group:

- All pivotal managers and department heads should be included on planning and design task force teams, as determined by the executive steering committee.

- General information sessions should be made mandatory for all managers and department heads.
- Every department manager even vaguely related to the chosen case types should attend the CareMap tool authoring sessions, *accompanied by* one of their staff members.
- The management group should be solicited for ratification of policies and procedures for both CareMap tool documentation and case management.
- The management group should be used to help design how variance data will be collected, aggregated, displayed, reviewed, and otherwise used.
- The management group should be used to redo performance appraisals and other related and reinforcing procedures.
- Managers should understand or have negotiated how the proposed changes will affect their own budgets. (It is important to remember that management is accountable for operationalizing programs.)

In summary, quality, financial, or political information should not be kept from the management group and the group should be involved at all phases. Figure 3-2 shows a well-tested progression of educational "waves" that support implementation of the project design.

Figure 3-2. Progression of Education for Outcome-Based Practice

I. Introduction (following consultation with administration by CCM)
(Approximately 1–2 hours long for all multidisciplinary staff and management)
   A. How is the health care industry changing?
      1. What does it mean for our agency?
      2. What are we going to do about it?
   B. What is a CareMap System and how does it fit into our plans?

II. CareMap Author Teams
   A. Write maps (2–4 hours)
   B. Be developed as team over 9–12 months

III. How to Use a CareMap Tool (2 hours)
   A. Use self-instruction learning before class
   B. Walk through case type during class

IV. Getting Comfortable with Variance (2 hours)
   A. Feelings about variance—discussion
   B. Variance as individualization and information
   C. What to do with variance
      1. Case consultation
      2. Health care team meetings

V. Clinical Management Skills for Outcome-Based Practice
   A. Critical thinking
   B. Inclusion
   C. Principled negotiation
   D. Follow-up and follow-through

Specialized Education

I. Patient population (or case type) specific update (4–8 hours)
   A. Anatomy & physiology
   B. Staying patient-centered
   C. Realistic and effective patient education
   D. Continuing care "beyond the walls"

II. Management/Department Head Skills
"Leading the Change to Outcome-based Practice"
Coaching

Source: Zander, K. *Progression of Education for Outcome-Based Practice.* South Natick, MA: The Center for Case Management, 1993. Used with permission.

The Program Infrastructure

Any organization striving to establish collaborative care as a program or a means to fit a mission must take it seriously enough to build a well-defined infrastructure. Ideally, this infrastructure would include a steering committee at the executive level, a full-time program manager/director, and collaborative self-managing teams. A case study presented at the end of this section illustrates how this infrastructure can work to advantage.

The Executive Steering Committee

The executive steering committee is the most important method for implementation of a collaborative care program. Its major function is to provide the program with knowledgeable direction and active leadership. In other words, the committee must oversee the collaborative care program, always evaluating its design and function against the organization's mission. Steering committees also neutralize turf issues and serve as models for collaborative care at the administrative level. This is an active, participative process that should last between three and five years or until collaborative care has been operationalized by management, whichever comes first.

Of note, the committee may be the same group, with a few additions, that already provides direction and authority to other programs within the organization. There is no need to have a completely separate collaborative care committee if the work can be integrated into the agenda of an already-established group.

If possible, the committee should include the organization's chief executive officer (CEO). It also should definitely include the following individuals:

- The chief information officer (or medical records, compiling services)
- The chief financial officer
- Formal physician leader or chief(s) of services
- Chief of patient care services (inpatient, ambulatory, home care)
- Vice-presidents or directors of quality assurance/utilization review/risk management, social services, pharmacy services, nutrition care, respiratory care, and physical therapy/occupational therapy
- Legal counsel as needed

The executive steering committee should meet monthly to keep implementation of the collaborative care program on target. Committee responsibilities include, but are not limited to:

- Reviewing, revising, and committing to a strategic plan with objectives, activities, target dates, responsible staff, and evaluation considerations; confirming the overall goals for establishing collaborative care
- Selecting institutional target case types and/or serving as a clearinghouse for selection, including LOS and cost per case, if possible
- Designating author teams for each target case type and providing them with education and information
- Reviewing and finalizing critical paths/CareMap tools that are submitted; approving a process by which these tools are typed, copied, and distributed
- Authorizing new systems to support collaborative care, such as intershift nursing report format and multidisciplinary discharge planning rounds
- Authorizing a mechanism for variance identification and analysis that meets the needs of CQI, utilization management, JCAHO requirements, and so on

Figure 3-3 shows the recommended infrastructure for implementation and maintenance of a collaborative care program until such time that it is totally integrated into everyday operations. As shown, the executive steering committee holds the "big picture" of mission and program, using the services of a full-time project manager to actualize the components of collaborative care.

In essence, the executive steering committee must continually answer questions such as the following:

- How important is this program to the mission of the hospital, and how much priority (financial, resources, involvement) will it receive?
- Who is authorized to make decisions about the different components of collaborative care?
- How will collaborative care dovetail, replace, subsume, and/or facilitate former, current, and anticipated endeavors?
- How can the committee ensure that this program is as inclusive of all levels and types of employees as possible, all the time?
- How can it ensure that practice decisions are always respected and not compromised for cost savings, egos, or politics?
- How will the committee communicate these changes internally and externally to the hospital's community, payers, competition, and so on?

The Project Manager

The appointment of a project manager probably is the single most important decision of the executive steering committee. The position may be shared but must be full-time if the organization is serious about collaborative care and wants to have it established relatively quickly. Typical project manager responsibilities are detailed at length in the case study documented at the end of this section.

To a large extent, the project manager uses an advisory group of managers, department heads, and selected clinicians to guide the collaborative care process and to problem-solve. This group also advises and actually teaches some of the information or skill modules necessary to the program. Members of the advisory group also may become facilitators of the multidisciplinary group that begins as CareMap authoring sessions and eventually becomes permanent clinical quality improvement teams. (The work of the author teams and format task forces shown in figure 3-3 is described in chapter 4.)

Figure 3-3. Recommended Infrastructure for Implementation and Maintenance of a Collaborative Care Program

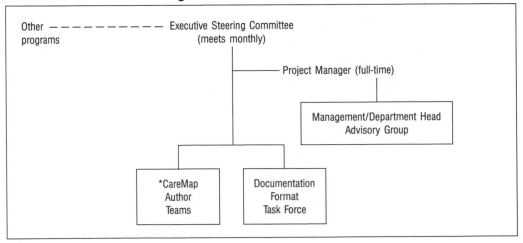

*Will become permanent groups

Collaborative Self-Managing Teams

A *self-managing team* is a team that has its own agenda, processes, goals, and ways to sustain itself through conflicts, external pressures, and easy times. As shown by Cog's Ladder model of group development in figure 3-4, a self-managing team is one that has achieved the *constructive stage* of group development.

Volumes have been written about self-managing teams in a multitude of settings. For the purpose of understanding the specific application to collaborative care, this section will focus on the types of teams necessary to conduct collaborative care and the preparation and support of those teams along a developmental framework.

Defining the Levels of Teams

There are roughly three levels of teams in collaborative care: direct-care teams, patient population (case type) teams, and program-level teams. (See figure 3-5.) *Direct-care teams* are composed of large numbers of people who are defined by the task to be done for a particular patient, rather than defined ahead of time as a formal team in which most or all members have worked together before and will work together again (for example, room teams, IV teams, nursing teams, and so on).

Patient population or case type teams are those defined by a larger category or assignment than one patient at a time. These teams are always multidisciplinary and should be formally appointed, educated, and facilitated. In collaborative care, these are the teams that initially author the CareMap tools and eventually—if encouraged, structured, and facilitated—become permanent teams that monitor outcomes and costs for care of a specific population or condition, such as congestive heart failure. Other examples might be the multidisciplinary geriatric assessment and treatment team, the liver transplant team, or the substance abuse team. These teams may include not only cross-area representatives but also cross-agency/community members.

Figure 3-4. The Cog's Ladder Model of Group Development

Phase	Characteristics	Movement
1. Polite possibility	Members need to be liked. Conflict absent. Polite conversation includes information sharing.	Phase 1 → 2.: Member must relinquish comfort and risk of conflict.
2. Why are we here?	Identity as a group still slow. Need to know goals and objectives. Cliques grow. Hidden agenda items begin to be sensed.	Phase 2 → 3: Must put aside discussion of group's purpose and commit to overall objectives which may not completely agree. Must risk personal attack.
3. Bid for power	Struggle for leadership occurs. No strong team spirit. Cliques most important. Wide range of participation by members. Need for structure strong.	Phase 3 → 4: Individuals must stop defending own views and risk possibility of being wrong. Requires humility. Can be blocked by strong member or clique. Members who don't move may be rejected.
4. Constructive	Team spirit starts to build. Individual talent used. Potential for creativity high.	Phase 4 → 5: Requires unanimous agreement. Demands trust. Risks breach of trust.
5. Esprit	High group morale. Intense group loyalty. Individuality and creativity high. Cliques absent. Group constructive and productive. Group strongly "closed." New member results in regression to earlier stage.	

Source: Charrier, G. Cog's Ladder: A model of group growth. In: Stone, S., and others, editors. *Management for Nurses: A Multidisciplinary Approach.* 3rd Ed. St. Louis: C. V. Mosby Co., 1984, pp. 104–10.

Figure 3-5. Levels of Teams in a Collaborative Care Program

Level	Function	Sample Membership
1. Individual patient	Give direct care and support services; use CareMap tools to document care, outcomes, and variances.	Dr. X, nurse Y, dietitian Z, plus lab, x-ray, respiratory therapy, secretaries, nursing staff assigned to patient around the clock, etc.
*2. Homogeneous population, case type	Author CareMap tools, track aggregate variance; recommend changes in system responses or practice patterns for specific population.	Author/clinical CQI teams: i.e., the CHF team. May include MD at chief or attending level, utilization review, expert people from each department and agency "servicing" CHF patients and their families.
*3. Program, product line	Review clinical and financial data for all patients within jurisdiction; recommend large system changes to achieve cost and quality goals; negotiate contracts.	Cardiac Centers co-directors, department leaders, case managers, data specialists, educators, etc.

*To be developed as self-managing teams

Program-level teams are composed of clinical and administrative leadership people. Their role is to develop and maintain a program of collaborative care at the level beyond case type, such as at the Cardiac Centers at Mercy and Unity Hospitals in Minneapolis. This structure is equivalent to a "product line" or "centers of excellence" structure. Another example might be pediatrics or pediatric orthopedics.

Like case type teams, program-level teams cross geographic boundaries. However, program-level teams would review practice and cost/quality data for a wider group of patients. They would also be more intensely involved in managed care contracting, organizational policies, and large system change. As shown in figure 3-5, some members of a group at one level also may belong to the group at the next level. This is a good way to tangibly link communication.

Because of the ad hoc nature of teams at the individual patient level, direct-care teams usually have neither the opportunity nor the desire to become self-managing (although this is not to say that each member should not conduct him- or herself as an autonomous individual). However, self-managing teams are most useful to the organization and most satisfying to their own members at the case type and program levels. At either level, the people in these newly defined groupings will not perceive a real team until they live experiences as a group. Therefore, they will likely need to be facilitated on a regular schedule through the proven stages of group growth.

Facilitating Collaborative Care Teams to Become Self-Managing Teams

Many organizations underestimate the importance of facilitation because the planners assume that intelligent, motivated professional people will automatically coalesce into a well-oiled group. In truth, all new groups benefit from a leader of some kind, especially at the beginning. A leader (facilitator) from the outside helps all members feel equal by lessening natural feelings of competition. Further, although groups must "work through" each phase of Cog's Ladder to reach the constructive phase, they will move faster with facilitation. The project manager or some other delegatee(s) may be a facilitator.

In addition to facilitation, collaborative care teams need a purpose. The collaborative care team development plan in figure 3-6 might be used as a sample to individualize care

Figure 3-6. Case Type Collaborative Care Team: Development Plan following CareMap Tool Authoring

Group Practice Name: _____

Facilitator: _____

Objectives	Activities	Staff	Target Date	Progress Reports

1. Complete creation of an initial case-type information packet for group	i. Integrate the CareMap tool across total episode of illness
	ii. Collect all relevant teaching materials
	iii. Collect and read case-related literature
	iv. Review standardized case management plans (as available) for total episode
	v. Other (examples):
	  • Protocols
	  • Flow sheets			

2. Establish/identify systems of communication among group members	i. Establish a meeting time and location ii. Establish a system for communicating with absent members iii. Agree upon the method for maintaining ongoing communication with all physician(s) (for example, rounds meeting) iv. Establish a method for maintaining information on the group's caseload (for example, a patient roster)			

3. Identify methods of admitting cases to the group practice	i. Identify how admission information will be obtained
	ii. Decide how cases will be admitted to the practice
	iii. Discuss if a case manager will be needed
	iv. Determine the meaning of "length of an episode" for the case type
	  • When does a case manager assume responsibility?
	  • How will patient telephone calls be handled (from patient)?
	  • What type of telephone calls will be made to the patient/by whom?
	v. Other			

4. Set quarterly goals relative to the management of the case type	i. Identify case-related learning needs
	ii. Other (examples):
	  • Assess targets of opportunity, given the current CareMap tool
	  • Integrate teaching plans/strategies across the episode of illness
	  • Evaluate/improve achievement of specific outcomes
	  • Reduce specific resource utilization if possible
	  • Review variances on critical path; make modifications as needed; identify needs for quality improvement
	  • Review systems of communication and make modifications as needed			

during and after the authoring of a critical path or CareMap document. Meetings of case type–level and product line–level teams need only occur quarterly once variance data become available. For a few meetings, the teams may need facilitation to help analyze the data because this is a relatively new skill for most clinicians.

The Cardiac Center of Mercy and Unity Hospitals represents an excellent example of a self-managing team at the product line level. The interdisciplinary representation is:

- Physicians
  - Internists
  - Intensivists
  - Cardiologists (chairperson, leader)
  - Pulmonologist
  - Anesthesiologist
  - Thoracic surgeons
  - Nurse clinicians
- Nursing (Line and Direct Nursing Supervisors)
  - OR
  - Intensive care unit (case managers)
  - Postcoronary care unit (case managers)
  - Cardiovascular case managers
  - Cardiology
- Department Representatives
  - Laboratory
  - Pharmacy
  - Respiratory therapy
  - Cardiac rehab
  - Home care
  - Quality management/medical records
  - Pastoral care/social service
  - Case management
  - Management information system
  - Financial services
- Administrative vice-president

This program has a fundamental self-managing cycle repeated quarterly throughout the year to handle cost and quality "business." The cycle includes:

- Month 1 – Review data as a multidisciplinary group
- Month 2 – Peer review (physicians only)
- Month 3 – Education for all

The centers collaboratively develop action plans to correct variances. Figure 3-7 shows 2 out of 10 such plans generated by this large self-managing team at the program level. Obviously, this is system-savvy collaborative care at its best, and demonstrates that clinicians can and will actively work on solutions to achieve cost and quality outcomes.

In conclusion, self-managing teams come in many forms yet have very definable development phases and a compelling need for facilitation. They are the heart of collaborative care and the logical goal of a highly decentralized organization. However, they will not succeed if they are not nurtured, empowered, listened to, and responded to. More important, if the motivated and talented professional staff do not believe they are taken seriously or that their concerns will be addressed readily by administration, they will quickly lose interest and cease participation in all aspects of collaborative care.

Figure 3-7.   Health One Mercy Hospital—CABG

Item #4
Person(s) responsible:

Proposed Action	Annual Cost Savings
Develop early discharge protocol to include home care visits.	• ↓ Cost by $100,000 → $200,000 • ↓ LOS by 1–2 days • Nurse time savings 6,000–10,000 hours

Major Activities	Person Responsible	Proposed Implementation Date	Quality Enhancements
1. Develop home care protocol for earlier discharge of selected patients. 2. Improved communication network between home care RNs and RN case managers, social services and nurse clinicians. 3. Early identification and assessment of this patient population. • Decision tree development 4. Monitor change in practice • Readmits • Home care audits • Hospital D/C audits	Joan McLean, RN Marilyn Siebel, MSW Sandy Pippo, RN Robin Uithoven, RN Mary Swander, RN Deb Curran, RN Bonnie Sentz, RN Sharon Henry, RN Karen Bowman, RN Peggy Bear, RN	8/92	1. Improved short-term outcomes. 2. Improved communication between patients and different groups of clinicians. 3. ↓ Readmissions. 4. Improved patient education.

Quantification Methodology

250 patients × 1 day = 250 days savings = 100,000
250 patients × 2 days = 500 days savings = 200,000

Source: Henry, S. Cardiac Centers, Health One Mercy Hospital, 1990. Used with permission.

Case Example of Program Infrastructure

A fine example of the establishment and ongoing work of an executive steering committee is found in Newton-Wellesley Hospital (NWH) in Newton, Massachusetts.[2] The hospital's reasons for planning a collaborative care project in 1991 and implementing it in 1992 were:

- To pursue a commitment to continuously improve the quality of patient care
- To support a concept uniquely suited to operationalizing many of the organization's five-year total quality management (TQM) goals to improve or enhance:
  - Patient care
  - Financial strength and stability
  - Leadership
  - Teaching
  - Employee commitment, motivation, and satisfaction
  - Medical staff
  - Facilities
  - Community relations
- To increase staff retention through staff recognition and satisfaction
- To provide clinical support for decision making and documentation
- To reduce LOS
- To reduce expenses and make more efficient use of resources
- To increase interdisciplinary collaboration (JCAHO requirement)
- To improve the potential to negotiate contracts with third-party payers

NWH's executive steering committee is composed of the following members:

- Director of rehab services
- Director of Newell Home Health

71

- Assistant vice-president for nursing
- Assistant vice-president for finance
- Director of nutrition services
- Director of outpatient services
- Nurse manager of 4 South
- Director of collaborative care project
- Director of medical records
- Director of laboratory services
- Vice-president for nursing
- Director of respiratory services
- Director of clinical information services
- Director of social services
- Director of pharmacy services
- Nurse manager of post-anesthesia care unit (PACU)
- Oncologist
- Director of QA/UR/risk management (RM)

Committee Responsibilities

Executive steering committee members have a number of crucial responsibilities. These include:

- To develop criteria for selection of case types for case management and to approve case types for inclusion in the collaborative care project
- To articulate the collaborative care project into the hospital's five-year TQM plan
- To review recommendations from group practices regarding changes in practice or policy and to make recommendations back to practice groups about the groups bringing changes to committees
- To serve the project manager in a consultative role when issues cannot be resolved by group practice members with the manager's assistance
- To review and recommend guidelines for the standardization of documentation (critical paths, CareMap tools)
- To approve standardized variance coding
- To evaluate the impact and outcomes of the collaborative care project, including:
  - Quality of care
  - Patient satisfaction
  - Project costs
  - Costs per case type
  - Staff satisfaction
  - Streamline documentation
- To make recommendations regarding the continuation, expansion, or termination of case management/managed care
- To receive and review periodic updates from group practices, including progress reports, minutes, and CareMap tools
- To receive and approve all group practice goals and outcome measures
- To establish ground rules for collaborative care, specifically with regard to:
  - Improving the quality of patient care
  - Improving patient satisfaction
  - Increasing multidisciplinary collaboration
  - Enhancing clinician satisfaction
  - Improving documentation systems
  - Providing high-quality care in a cost-effective manner

To that end, five case types were selected. These were:

1. HEAL (Help educate after loop) patients
2. Depressed patients receiving electroconvulsive therapy (ECT)
3. Uncomplicated myocardial infarction (MI) patients
4. Total hip replacement patients
5. Acute myelogenous leukemia (AML) patients

Once the case types were chosen, the members of each collaborative care team could be recommended. (See figure 3-8.)

In time, NWH created a one-person collaborative care department (with a budget). Creation of a collaborative care department is recommended only when a strong, committed steering committee exists; otherwise the program will suffer from lack of interest and ownership by those not in the designated department. Although at NWH the project manager reports to the assistant vice-president of nursing (AVPN), the AVPN is on the committee through long-standing credibility and has a major influence in the organization.

Project Manager Responsibilities

The project manager has overall responsibility for coordinating the planning, implementation, and evaluation of the multidisciplinary collaborative care project at NWH. In collaboration with the steering committee, he or she:

* Oversees the ongoing development of implementation strategies, orientation, and education about case management concepts to medical, nursing, and other health care professionals; provides ongoing evaluation of the project outcomes; and establishes collaborative care practice teams

Figure 3-8. Newton-Wellesley Hospital Collaborative Care Group Practice Members

MI

Cardiologist
RN—ED
RN—CCU
RN—3W
Nutrition
Pharmacy
Physical therapist
Cardiovascular rehab
Laboratory—Chemistry Dept.
Cardiac diagnostics
EKG

HEAL

Obstetrician
Social worker
RN—ED
RNs—5W
RN—day surgery
Ultrasound
Admitting
Clergy
Childbirth Education
Clinical leader—SCNN
RN—Labor and Delivery
Clinical leader—maternal

Total Hip

Orthopedic surgeon
RN—Henderson Building
  (outpatient)
RN—Operating Room
RN—4 West
Cont. care nurse
Nutrition
Physical therapist
Social service

AML Leukemia

Oncologist
RN—4 South
RN—oncology
Nutrition
Pharmacist
IV therapy RN
Social service
Laboratory—Blood Bank
Physical therapy
RN-Newell Home Health
Infectious disease RN

Depression with ECT Therapy

Psychiatrist
Anesthesiologist
RN—Usen 3
RN—3 East
RN—PACU
Social service
Psych OT

- Effectively communicates and integrates the mission, values, and strategic initiatives of the hospital
- Demonstrates behaviors consistent with the CQI process
- Participates on hospitalwide committees and task forces, communicating and collaborating with both managers and employees

Recognized as having a management leadership position within the hospital organization, the project manager utilizes the hospital's policies, procedures, and other resources in the performance of his or her activities and responsibilities. Additionally, he or she assumes responsibility for maintaining his or her own professional education. (See figure 3-9 for NWH project manager qualifications and responsibilities.)

Figure 3-9. NWH Collaborative Care Project Manager: Summary of Major Areas of Performance

Responsibilities:

1. Assumes the chairperson responsibilities for the Collaborative Care Steering Committee.

2. Regularly provides communication and feedback to the Steering Committee about the progress of the practice groups.

3. Recommends to the Steering Committee criteria for selection of case types and long-term practice group member complement for specific case types.

4. In collaboration with the Steering Committee, defines project goals that articulate into the Focus 95 plan.

5. Develops systems to both monitor and evaluate the achievement of project goals.

6. Seeks advice from the Steering Committee about the resolution of issues which cannot be resolved at the group practice level.

7. Supports the formation of Collaborative Care Practice Groups, including the development and ongoing evaluation of the strategic plans for implementation of each case type.

8. In collaboration with practice group members, establishes overall practice group goals, objectives, activities, and target dates that are consistent with overall project goals.

9. Plans for, leads, and participates in regularly scheduled meetings of the CC practice groups. Facilitates group members acquiring increased independence in these responsibilities.

10. Supports the Collaborative Practice Groups by serving as a resource to provide assistance and expertise in: development of critical path content, establishing baseline information on case types, acquiring information about hospital systems, evaluating group progress, and negotiating problem solving for issues which cannot be resolved at the group practice level.

11. Guidelines and support plans for the continuous assessment of the quality of patient care and its impact on patient care outcomes. Facilitates group members acquiring increased independence in these responsibilities.

12. Facilitates communication between practice groups and hospital departments, managers, and hospital committees about improvement opportunities.

13. Supports the analysis of the level of patient satisfaction by group members through use of hospital satisfaction surveys.

14. Maintains and acquires knowledge of patient care needs for patient populations in the Collaborative Care Project.

15. Interacts and intervenes with appropriate members of hospital staff for purposes of assessing the care provided.

16. Identifies appropriate resources within the institution to provide consultation, education, technical or informational services as needed for self, practice group members, or patients.

17. Maintains close working relationships with managers and staff whose departments provide support services to patients in the CC Project. Initiates and/or facilitates appropriate communications and planning to ensure a consistently high level of service to the CC patients and to effectively meet any special needs of the patients in the CC Project and other patients in the hospital.

18. Analyzes the level of staff satisfaction among members of the practice groups.

Documentation Task Force Responsibilities

A documentation subcommittee (task force) was appointed whose major responsibility was to go beyond the format of CareMap tools to examine major multidisciplinary conceptual, regulatory, and information needs. The subcommittee's short- and long-term objectives were to streamline documentation systems (potentially to the level of "documentation by exception"), automate documentation systems, integrate the medical record (which is patient rather than discipline oriented), and demonstrate interdisciplinary collaboration. Its considerations were to understand current charting policies, individual discipline standards, JCAHO requirements, and the educational needs of clinicians using the record. Task force members included some steering committee members along with appropriate experts such as the director of clinical computing.

Figure 3-9. (Continued)

19. Facilitates ongoing professional development of group practice members.

20. Assists in the development of a care delivery system consistent with changes in patient needs, medical technology, and the professions involved with specific case types.

21. Makes suggestions for improved work processes within the scope of the project.

22. Coordinates the development and evolution of the Collaborative Care documentation system including critical paths, variation tracking, and the integrated progress note that focuses on a coordinated, streamlined, complete multidisciplinary view of the patient's progress.

23. Guides practice groups in the content development of critical paths which will ultimately yield ongoing patient-specific and aggregate data related to patient outcome, quality and appropriateness of care, and opportunities for improvement.

24. Facilitates the development and implementation of a system of variation tracking to monitor the care of CC patients and assists group members in the analysis of aggregate variation data.

25. Evaluates and makes recommendations about Collaborative Care Documentation systems in relation to current and anticipated documentation and QA systems.

26. Develops and presents the curriculum for orientation and education regarding collaborative care to medical, nursing, and other health care professionals within the designated practice groups.

27. Establishes formal and informal educational sessions for current staff and oversees the incorporation of Collaborative Care into the orientation program for new staff.

28. Coordinates response to external requests for presentation, site visits, and consultation.

29. Is a resource for all staff regarding Collaborative Care. Provides consultation to all other areas which can utilize his/her expertise.

30. Participates on nursing and hospital committees.

31. Develops proposals of budgetary needs and submits to AVPN. Responsible for operating within approved budget or justifying variances.

Qualifications:

1. Master's-prepared clinician.

2. Strong leadership skills and previous management experience including experience in facilitating interdisciplinary collaboration. Evidence of this should include:

   a. Effective communication skills
   b. Ability to deal well with people
   c. Ability to problem-solve
   d. Ability to appropriately confront issues
   e. Ability to motivate others as individuals and as a group
   f. Ability to plan, organize, and direct the activities of others

3. Previous project implementation preferred.

The task force made a number of important recommendations in information sheets such as the one shown in figure 3-10. Similar kinds of information sheets in collaborative care programs around the world look deceptively simple. However, they do describe the "guts" of a new system and provide users from every discipline with answers to their questions and concerns.

Along those same lines, the NWH steering committee grew to understand and direct the concept of variance. Members agreed that there would always be variation in both patient outcomes and interventions, and saw critical path maps as a way to "monitor care and evaluate the appropriateness of interventions in relation to patient outcomes." They proposed added precision to the standard variance identification with the following categories:

- Negative variance for intervention—no effect on outcome
- Negative variance for intervention—negative outcome
- Negative variance for intervention—positive outcome
- Positive variance for intervention—no effect on outcome
- Positive variance for intervention—negative outcome
- Positive variance for intervention—positive outcome

Figure 3-11 traces the evolution of typical themes and dilemmas over the first several years of collaborative care at NWH. The issues outlined in the figure were addressed by the steering committee as it successfully built a collaborative care program.

Case Studies

This section studies collaborative care program design issues addressed by three types of hospitals: a regional hospital, a community teaching hospital, and a medical center. Despite obvious differences in size and location, all three have much in common and continue to have strong collaborative care programs.

Case Study 1. The Regional Hospital

Lakes Region General Hospital (LRGH) is a 143-bed, not-for-profit, acute care regional hospital located in Laconia, New Hampshire. As a level III trauma center and designated rural referral center, LRGH provides general and specialized health care services to the communities of the state's lake and mountain regions. Through a variety of strategies, LRGH has fulfilled its mission of collaborative care on several levels, recently acknowledged by the inaugural NOVA Awards for collaboration from the American Hospital Association (AHA) and *Hospitals and Health Networks.*[3]

The initial LRGH mission statement specifies health services that are appropriate and delivered in a financially responsible manner, all the while being assessed for ways to improve. It is planned that a revised mission statement will include the goals of promoting health status and well-being, as well as the integration rather than duplication of services between LRGH and community agencies. To meet the mission set by the hospital's strategic planning committee (which includes the board), a network of delivery system components woven together through a CQI framework, as shown in figure 3-12, has been creatively designed. Essentially, LRGH is using a growing number of multidisciplinary CareMap tools, with primary nursing on each unit and continuous clinical improvement teams to review care across units; care management for selected populations; and case management for the HealthLink (uninsured) population.

Figure 3-10. Forms Justification Sheet: Critical Path and Integrated Progress Note

Purpose of New Form

The multidisciplinary "Critical Path" format is an integral part of the documentation system designed for use with Collaborative Care project patients. This documentation system is intended to streamline and improve both the quality and completeness of documentation by all disciplines involved in the patient's care. Additionally, this system will ultimately yield data for ongoing quality assessment/improvement activities as a by-product of patient documentation, rather than as a separate, retrospective QA activity. The general format submitted for approval will be trialed for each of the five case types currently in the project; the specific preprinted content will vary for each of the case types.

The critical path maps expected patient progress over the entire episode of illness. The path represents a picture of the standard of "average" patient; it is not a substitute for physician's orders. Individualization to the specific patient is intended. Expected patient outcomes and the interventions necessary to achieve them are listed and documented against. Through this mapping, clinicians are able to see the expected progress and relationship of interventions to outcomes. A primary goal of this documentation system is to understand how different interventions affect patient outcomes. Analysis of variation data will provide us with information about areas in which we do well and areas needing improvement.

How Is This Information Currently Documented? How Is This Documentation Inadequate?

The information is currently documented in each discipline's separate progress note and/or flowsheets. Comprehensive documentation of care provided is frequently found to be lacking, from the perspective of standards of practice or regulatory/review agencies. The discipline providing care is the central organizing focus of our current charting systems; critical paths will focus instead on a coordinated, multidisciplinary view of the patient's progress.

Will This Form Be Replacing Any Form(s) Currently in Use?

Separate progress notes for each of the disciplines involved will be replaced by a single integrated, patient-focused progress note. In addition, the activity flowsheet for Nursing will be eliminated for these patients.

Who Will Complete This New Form?

The integrated progress note will be completed by all disciplines caring for patients of the Collaborative Care Project.

What Kinds of Problems Will This Form Help Solve for Your Area?

Increase coordinated, centralized communication between disciplines and decrease duplication. Make very apparent areas where patients are not progressing as expected so that timely interventions can be instituted. Improve completeness of information in the record. Decrease time required for narrative charting of routine, repetitive, expected information.

Will This Form Be a Part of the Permanent Medical Record?

Yes.

Are There Any External Requirements for This Form? (i.e. JCAHO)

Two major focuses of the current JCAHO standards require:

- Evidence of the collaborative effort between disciplines in planning, delivering, and evaluating patient care
- Patient outcome focus in documentation and evaluation of care

These focuses reflect the primary goals of the Collaborative Care project and the documentation formats proposed.

Medical Records Form: If This Form Is a Checklist or a Flowchart, Have Other Alternatives Been Explored?

The critical path documentation system is viewed by the Collaborative Care project as a:

- Teaching tool, which guides staff in planning, delivering, and evaluating patient care
- Guide to comprehensive care, which maintains the opportunity for individualizing care to the specific patient
- Streamlined documentation format, which frees the clinician from detailed narrative documentation of routine, expected, repetitive aspects of patient care
- CQI (continuous quality improvement) tool, which yields ongoing patient-specific and aggregate data related to patient outcome, quality and appropriateness of care, and opportunities for improvement

The advantages and disadvantages of preprinted formats against which care is charted have been explored extensively by the Collaborative Care Steering Committee, Documentation Task Force, and practice groups. It is felt that the advantages to be derived (as listed above) offer the opportunity for significant improvement in the current quality of documentation in the medical record, as well as in interdisciplinary collaboration, and QA/QI follow-up.

Source: Griffin, D. Newton-Wellesley Hospital. Used with permission.

Figure 3-11. Newton-Wellesley Time Line (in Retrospect)

April 1991:	Steering committee formed; five case types selected for specific reasons; implementation plan and project evaluation proposed
June 1991:	Variance coding discussed
July 1991:	Steering Committee *itself* tries its hand at variance coding to work out a system that will give them new, important information
August 1991:	Discuss problem of accuracy of length of stay statistics; discuss means to be consistent
September 1991:	Pilot project evaluation criteria adjusted; MD involvement discussed
October 1991:	Appoint documentation subcommittee to look at total medical record integration
November 1991:	Continue to discuss role of Steering Committee
December 1991:	Take on challenge of how to measure patient and staff satisfaction; appoint subcommittees
April 1992:	Final version of CareMap document approved by medical record
March 1992:	Discussion of whether to and how to tell patients they are in Collaborative Care program
June 1992:	Steering Committee *itself* composes a draft introductory letter to patients in Collaborative Care, elaborated upon by the Orthopedic Collaborative Practice Group
July 1992:	Discussions about how to really measure improvements in the quality of care, as well as the operational issue of how to identify Collaborative Care patients on the chart, etc.
September 1992:	First Collaborative Care patient admitted!
December 1992:	Patient satisfaction scores received
1993 and 1994:	Steering Committee continues to meet twice a month to discuss: • New case types • Ongoing evaluation of all parameters • Methods to continuously support Collaborative Care

Compiled from minutes of steering committee, Newton-Wellesley Hospital. Used with permission.

CareMap Tools

In his report on the medical staff, the chief of staff pointed to two changes in the delivery of high-quality care: The first is replacement of medical staff committees with multidisciplinary issue-related quality improvement teams, and the second involves CareMap tools developed according to practice guidelines. "The object is to treat patients with similar diagnoses in a similar manner. This approach allows consolidation of services and efficient planning of the hospital's resources, with the result of providing the highest quality of care in the optimal time at minimal costs."[4]

In 1992, a CareMap steering committee was established to support the author groups, coordinate staff and patient education on the CareMap system, monitor and direct the program's overall development and acceptable standardization program, and ensure the usefulness and clarity of the data generated, including future automation. Twenty-eight CareMap tools are in use or development, beginning with acute MI, transurethral resection of the prostate (TUR-P), and followed by chronic obstructive pulmonary disease (COPD), vaginal delivery, cesarean section, newborn, total hip replacement, total knee replacement, respiratory failure/ventilator, pneumonia, diabetes, congestive heart failure (CHF), renal, terminal, depression, anxiety, confusion, psychosis, laminectomy, upper abdominal surgery, hysterectomy, and tonsillectomy and adenoidectomy.

Of special note are the CareMap tools developed between emergency services and other constituencies. These include asthma and thrombolytic therapy, as well as the even more complex service-coordinating case types of suicide attempt/ideation and child abuse. The collaborative suicide team includes:

- The city prosecutor
- The Laconia Police Department

- Emergency department (ED) and ICU nurses and physicians
- A psychiatrist
- Lakes Regional Mental Health
- Behavioral health sciences clinicians
- Security

The suicide team used a facilitator, case critiques, a current flowchart, and each discipline's perspective to develop the CareMap tools for the ED and ICU. It was found that as the first issue of confidentiality emerged, the system in place to protect confidentiality and patient rights ended up contributing to the fragmentation of care.[5] With legal input from the prosecutor, victim/witness coordinators, and others, the team worked through the old intra-agency issues and decided that information directly relevant to a patient's treatment at each stage could be shared.

LRGH is using the same collaborative information analysis and CareMap development process with the child abuse team. This team is composed of:

- Division of Children, Youth and Families (DCYF)
- The Laconia Police Department
- The Belknap County victim witness coordinator
- An ED physician and nurse
- A pediatrician
- A county health service nurse
- The director of CQI
- The director of risk management

Figure 3-12. Enhanced Delivery System: Key Components

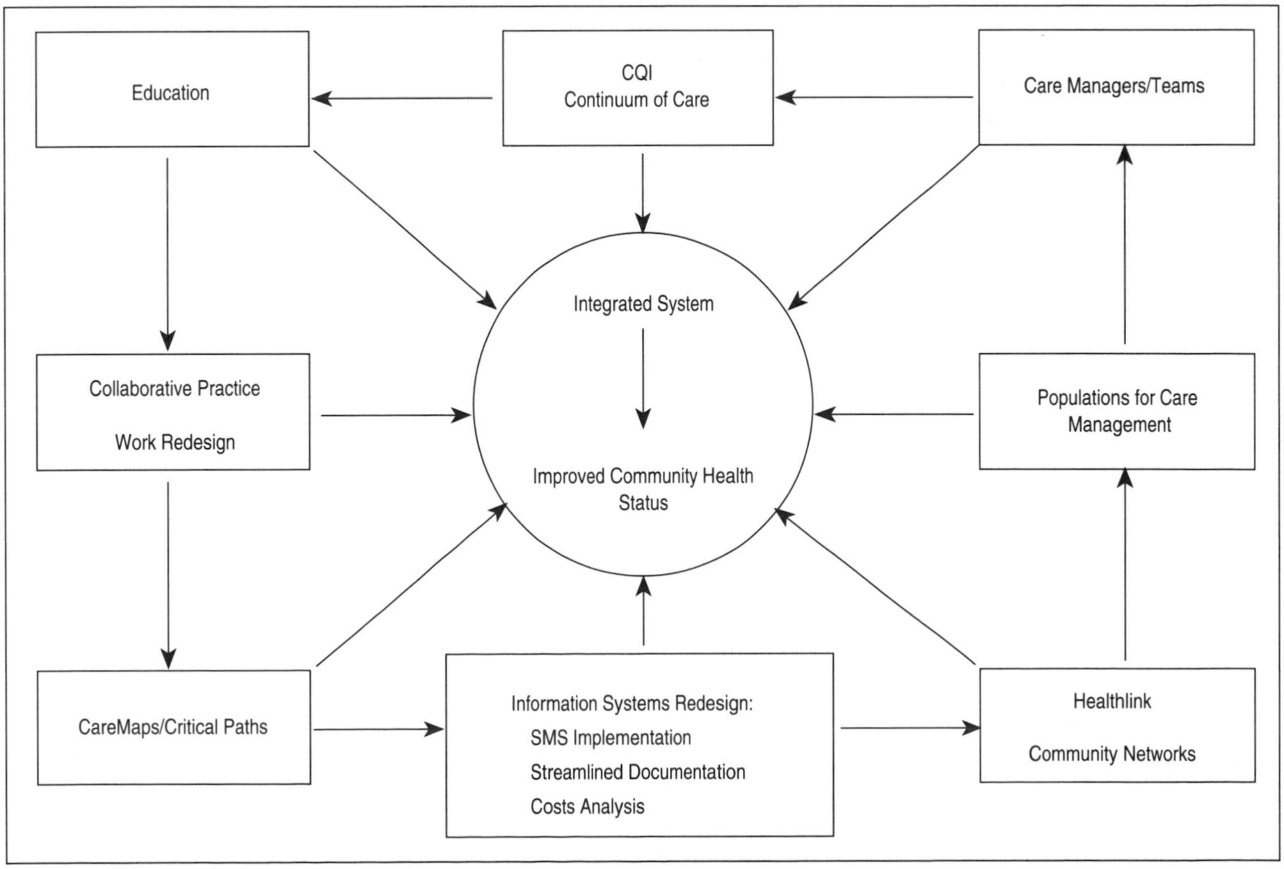

Reprinted, with permission, from Lakes Regional General Hospital, Laconia, NH. Used with permission.

With the energy and commitment behind such collaborative endeavors, LRGH undoubtedly will continue to extend its delivery system with new projects of mapping care for outpatient detox and geriatric dementia patients.

Additionally, beneath LRGH's success is a commitment to accurate information systems. The hospital's vice-president for professional services and finances states:

> As part of an organizationwide effort to favorably affect profitability, department directors identified initiatives to improve operational productivity. Clinical practice productivity opportunities, which include increasing quality, improving outcomes, standardizing care, and affecting utilization, were the largest category in potential dollars. The use of CareMap tools, linked with cost information, appears to be one of the key vehicles for realizing the opportunities available to Lakes Region General Hospital. Cost information is essential to maintaining physician interest and participation in care mapping."[6]

Care Management

LRGH clearly sees how information underlies care management. Care managers provide information at various stages of the patient's hospital stay that can be used to improve patient care while in the hospital and at home, as well as to improve the care process. Figure 3-13 shows the principal stages of the patient processing system and lists opportunities for improvement.

LRGH uses care managers to focus coordination on nonpatternable or complex, high-risk patient populations. Care managers are clinical II or III level staff nurses who come from the unit nursing budget but whose coordination of care may extend beyond their unit. Some of their patients have CareMap tools, and some may or may not have had major *detours* (the LRGH term for variances) in their clinical course.

Figure 3-13. Patient Processing System

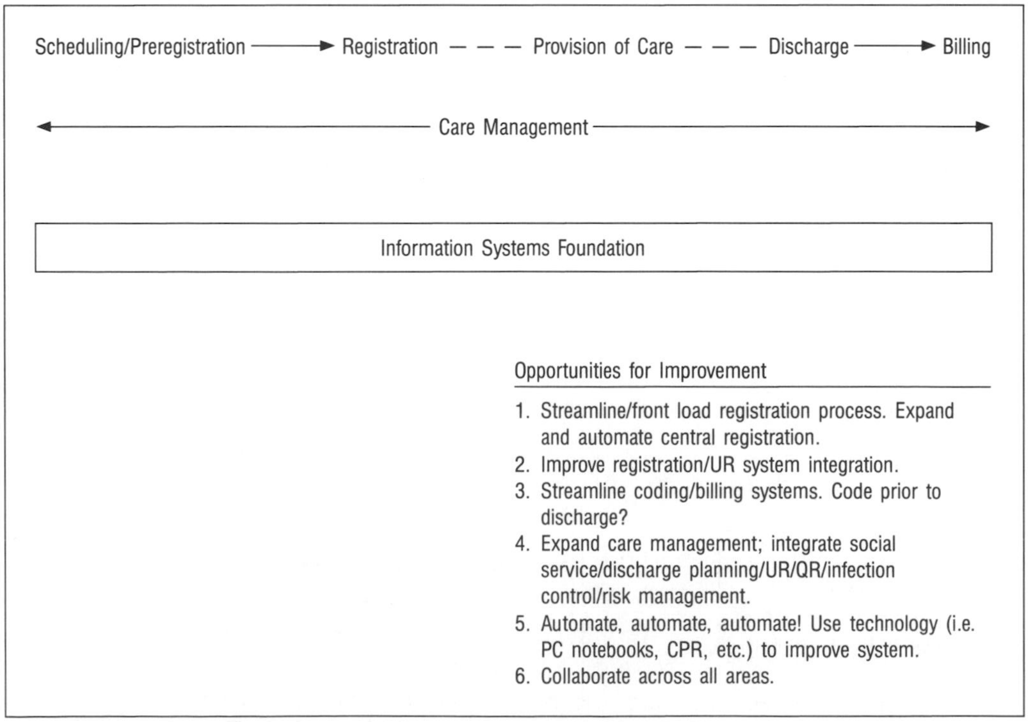

Skrajewski, D. Patient Processing System, 12/6/93. Used with permission.

Client criteria for a pilot continuing care management program include:

- Patient not managed by other service agency on admission
- Complicated medical needs
- Multiple medical diagnosis
- Patient not eligible for community services or not home bound
- Multiple recent readmissions
- History of noncompliance
- Nonpatternable patient

The care manager's responsibilities are many and varied. These include:

- To collaborate with quality review to ensure that the patient's care placed on the appropriate map
- To provide a well-coordinated care experience for patients and families
- To promote continuity of plan via the CareMap tool
- To identify anticipated discharge medications in collaboration with members of the health care team, with particular attention to normal routine and care-giving responsibilities (if any) at home
- To identify complex patients, referring to the continuing care management team for assessment
- To review medical record at discharge to assess patient's educational needs, activities, and discharge orders
- To follow up with a phone call within 48 hours to view survival skills, activity, safety, home care, proper administration of medication, and so on
- To analyze data to identify trends in variance and to share the data with the CareMap group to make effective change

HealthLink

Begun in 1994, HealthLink emerged from LRGH's strong sense of community responsibility to proactively address the area's health needs. It enrolls 300 people a month who are ineligible for Medicare or Medicaid benefits but qualify under HealthLink's criteria. Services are donated (LRGH absorbing $1 million to $1.5 million annually) by 77 health care providers and agencies within the region. Blue Cross/Blue Shield of New Hampshire provides actuarial support. Federal funds provide prescription drug benefits.[7]

To ensure that care is managed, HealthLink plans to use a third-generation case management model that calls for an up-front health and risk assessment, extensive patient education, outcomes measurement, and counseling. The model aims to make patients more self-sufficient on health matters and aware of the costs and consequences of unhealthy life-styles and behaviors.

LRGH is responding to the fluid nature of the health care industry within a larger changing society by using dynamic yet precise infrastructures. It is vigorously taking on the concerns of the elderly in the community, as well as the nature of chronic illness and other problems causing suffering and readmissions. CareMap tools, collaborative continuous clinical improvement groups, care management, and case management are the infrastructures LRGH has chosen not as ends in themselves but, rather, as a way to stay flexible and responsive.

Case Study 2. The Community Teaching Hospital

The Miriam Hospital is a 247-bed teaching hospital located in Providence, Rhode Island. The patient population is adult medical–surgical, and Medicare comprises more than 50 percent of annual admissions (11,373 patients in 1993). Primary nursing is the practice model for the nursing department.

In 1988, the Miriam Hospital was experiencing the full financial impact of Medicare's prospective payment system. Excessive LOS combined with consistently high-occupancy rates were resulting in frequent cancellation of admissions. All these elements created a potentially dire situation for the hospital's survival. An LOS task force composed of the clinical and administrative leadership was formed to identify strategies to reduce LOS and maximize capacity. Three tactics were identified and implemented: (1) a 9 a.m. discharge policy, (2) a short-stay surgical program, and (3) a pilot project utilizing critical paths.

The critical path pilot program implemented was modeled on the New England Medical Center's (NEMC's) pioneer work in the mid-1980s. Care management using critical paths appeared to be a viable way to address the hospital's LOS crisis without requiring either staff reductions or a decrease in other patient care resources. With the recommendations and support of the LOS task force, the critical path program was endorsed by the hospital's medical staff executive committee and the board of directors.

The primary goal of the initial pilot program was to decrease LOS without negatively affecting quality of care. The task force chose the initial two populations: coronary artery bypass graft (CABG) surgery and acute myocardial infarction (AMI) patients. Although no specific time frame for implementation was designated, the urgency of reducing hospitalization days was conveyed.

The Pilot Project

Miriam's vice-president for patient services, including nursing service, assumed primary responsibility for implementing the critical path pilot project. The assistant nurse-in-chief for special care was selected as project director. After a two-day education session at NEMC, the project director developed a four-month pilot plan with a six-week design phase, eight weeks of clinical implementation, and two weeks for evaluation.

Although the LOS task force monitored the initial pilot results, a pilot planning committee, composed primarily of nurse managers, designed the specifics of the project. Both the CABG and AMI critical paths were created collaboratively by multidisciplinary teams of practitioners caring for these patient populations. Support from the physician-in-chief and the surgeon-in-chief facilitated physician participation in the development of these initial paths.

During the six-week design phase, the project director's efforts were directed to tool structure, content, usage guidelines, communication with key medical staff, and education of appropriate clinical staff. Path design and content sessions took place over four weeks and provided an opportunity to teach program concepts to the health team members as well as gain project support. Communication with the 20 medical staff members whose patients would be involved in the pilot was extremely time-consuming but a leading factor in gaining path acceptance. Staff education was provided for all caregivers in the six clinical areas that would be caring for these patients. Education sessions focused primarily on documentation issues and were provided "just in time" for pilot implementation.

Evaluation of the pilot project was based primarily on the goal of reducing LOS for these two patient groups. After eight weeks of clinical implementation, the average LOS went from 8.9 to 5.9 days for AMI patients and from 12.7 to 10.2 days for CABG patients. Additionally, informal surveys of the medical and nursing staffs produced positive comments concerning the capacity of variance analysis to produce system changes for long-term problems and the clinical relevance of the paths. Staff also expressed concerns with double documentation, "policing" physician practice, and fostering "cookbook" medicine. Based on the dramatic reductions in LOS with the pilot, the critical path project was expanded to include the next leading patient groups at the hospital.

Project Expansion

Over the next two years, the number of paths increased to 31 and the positive impact on average LOS was sustained. Monitoring and analysis of pathway variance resulted in significant changes in hospital operations and improved patient care practices. (See figure 3-14.) The cost saving in terms of reduced patient days was estimated between $1.5 and $1.8 million. Decreased resource consumption also was demonstrated in a number of patient groups that were managed via critical paths. (See figure 3-15.)

Figure 3-14. Care Management and Case Management: Improvement Measures

Quality Measures—Changes in Practices/Systems:

- Increase in thallium stress testing slots
- Policy change related to obtaining sputum specimens
- Early morning reporting of enzyme results
- Revision of cardiology patient teaching program
- Nursing and admitting meeting—daily
- Pilot project for "fast-tracking" open-heart patients
- Patient satisfaction survey results
- Quarterly or biannual review of clinical practice guidelines

Source: McKenna, M. The Miriam Hospital. Used with permission.

Figure 3-15. Care Management and Case Management: Resource Consumption

DRG #107

Year	Vol.	Avg. LOS	Tot. $	Avg. Margin	Lab Units	Imaging Units	Therapy Units
1988	94.0	12.7	11700.0	4605.0	178.4	8.4	89.4
1989	125.0	11.4	12373.0	5240.0	153.0	7.8	72.3
1990	146.0	10.3	12937.0	4424.0	132.9	7.0	64.7
1991	144.0	10.7	12867.0	5902.0	160.2	7.0	51.1
1992	242.0	10.8	13467.0	7479.0	185.1	8.4	56.8

DRG #112

Year	Vol.	Avg. LOS	Tot. $	Avg. Margin	Lab Units	Imaging Units	Therapy Units
1988	193.0	7.1	5480.0	409.0	62.6	1.7	5.3
1989	304.0	5.9	4819.0	939.0	57.1	1.4	5.0
1990	389.0	5.2	5419.0	979.0	56.4	1.5	2.9
1991	407.0	5.1	6045.0	420.0	57.2	1.0	2.4
1992	480.0	4.4	6672.0	693.0	52.0	.82	2.2

DRG #140

Year	Vol.	Avg. LOS	Tot. $	Avg. Margin	Lab Units	Imaging Units	Therapy Units
1988	267.0	5.1	2451.0	22.0	43.0	1.9	4.9
1989	281.0	4.5	2178.0	166.0	40.6	1.6	2.4
1990	322.0	4.4	2541.0	−133.0	38.7	1.6	2.8
1991	289.0	4.3	2771.0	−3810.0	39.5	1.8	3.8
1992	309.0	3.8	2464.0	72.0	37.6	2.2	3.4

DRG #209

Year	Vol.	Avg. LOS	Tot. $	Avg. Margin	Lab Units	Imaging Units	Therapy Units
1988	152.0	12.9	8924.0	−210.0	55.8	2.2	40.4
1989	173.0	12.5	10708.0	−497.0	63.2	2.5	83.7
1990	190.0	10.9	10420.0	−327.0	56.0	2.2	62.7
1991	219.0	10.6	11152.0	−573.0	60.8	2.4	30.1
1992	216.0	9.3	11389.0	−144.0	53.2	2.2	28.0

Source: CQMS Reports. Reprinted with permission.

Nursing practice at the Miriam Hospital was greatly influenced by the renewed emphasis that critical paths place on the daily management and coordination of patient care services. It was at the suggestion of nursing staff that the patient-outcome-focused nursing care plans were developed to complement the process-oriented paths. The simplicity, logic, and appropriateness of using these CareMap-like tools to measure and evaluate nursing practice were recognized. Using the attainment of specific patient discharge outcomes as the quality measure for professional interventions, nursing discharge audits were developed. (See figure 3-16.) These have become a cornerstone in the unit-based quality improvement plans.

Initiation of the Nurse Case Manager Role

The role of the nurse case manager began to evolve in 1990 with recognition that some patients' hospitalizations were so variable that they could not be adequately managed solely with the use of a critical path/CareMap tool. Concurrently, it was acknowledged that the hospital's clinical advancement program was no longer meeting the needs of the expert nursing practitioner who wished to remain at the bedside. Nursing leadership decided that the nurse case manager role would address both these issues.

Over the ensuing nine-month period, the nursing department's philosophy of practice, primary nursing model, position descriptions, performance appraisal tools, and salary ranges were reviewed and modified to support this new clinical position. Education sessions were held for all members of the nursing department and other health team members. Additionally, a formal case management program was developed and presented to potential candidates. Selection of the case types to be case-managed was based on patient volume and complexity of care. The first three cardiology case managers assumed their roles in January 1991.

The Response to Organizational Needs

Rapid changes continued in all aspects of the critical path/CareMap tool and case management programs. The original critical paths have been totally redesigned and incorporated into the permanent medical record. Aggregate variance reporting is conducted monthly and serves as a basis for evaluating care on both a clinical and administrative level.

Critical path/CareMap tool and case management systems also have found an appropriate "fit" with a newly adopted TQM philosophy: The creation and daily utilization of the critical path/CareMap tool is the clinical application of Shewhart/Deming's plan-do-check-act (PDCA) improvement cycle.[8] Case managers use the similar CQI processes in the daily planning and modification of their goal-directed patient care activities.

In 1993, the impact of daily clinical management and decision making became more accurately reflected in bottom-line financial reports and national quality indicator surveys. The hospital's leadership groups typically sought assistance through critical path/CareMap tools or the expertise of nurse case managers in defining and/or monitoring the cost-effectiveness and efficiency of patient care services.

New outcome measures to indicate the nurse case managers' impact on the quality of care were patient satisfaction surveys and readmission rates. Case-managed patients at the Miriam Hospital have consistently rated their hospital experiences more positively than the national mean. (See figure 3-17.) The monthly unplanned readmission rate for case-managed patients is now less than 4 percent. All readmissions within 31 days are reviewed to assess discharge status and adequacy of the post-hospitalization plan.

Figure 3-16. The Miriam Hospital Case Management AMI Patient Outcome Audit Tool, DRG 122

	Follow-up plan/referral
Guidelines:	

Guidelines:

—Audit to be completed by registered nurse caregiver
—Audit to be completed the day of discharge or the day before discharge
—All items *must* have yes or no answer
—All negative responses *require* follow-up plan and/or referral

Chart Data

Kardex/continued note/and/or flowsheet address:

a. Patient's breath sounds are clear or have returned to baseline. Yes _____ No _____

b. Patient has no peripheral edema or has returned to baseline. Yes _____ No _____

c. Cardiac rhythm is stable or pulse and BP are within normal limits for the patient. Yes _____ No _____

Observation Data

"Can the patient ambulate 30 feet without developing:"

a. Cardiac discomfort? Yes _____ No _____

b. Dizziness? Yes _____ No _____

c. S.O.B.? Yes _____ No _____

Patient Interview Data

Say to the patient: "Tell me, what would you do if you have cardiac discomfort?"

a. Rest Yes _____ No _____

b. Take NTG Yes _____ No _____

c. Call EMS (911) Yes _____ No _____

"Have all your questions and concerns been addressed while you have been here?" Yes _____ No _____

"What type of activity should you do when you go home?"

a. Gradually increase activity (walking) Yes _____ No _____

b. Rest when tired Yes _____ No _____

"What activities shouldn't you do?"

a. Heavy lifting Yes _____ No _____

b. Driving Yes _____ No _____

"Do you have any of the following risk factors? If yes, what is your plan?"

Smoking Yes _____ No _____ Plan _____

High blood pressure Yes _____ No _____ Plan _____

High cholesterol Yes _____ No _____ Plan _____

Obesity Yes _____ No _____ Plan _____

Sedentary lifestyle Yes _____ No _____ Plan _____

Diabetes Yes _____ No _____ Plan _____

Stress Yes _____ No _____ Plan _____

Choose one medication that the patient will take at home and ask:

a. What medication is for. Yes _____ No _____

b. How often to take/day. Yes _____ No _____

c. Time of day to take medication. Yes _____ No _____

"When is your appointment with your doctor?" Patient gives a date/time period. Yes _____ No _____

"Have you considered attending a cardiac rehabilitation program?" Yes _____ No _____

RN signature _____

Date _____

7/92
Rev. 11/93

Source: The Miriam Hospital. Used with permission.

Figure 3-17. The Miriam Hospital Patient Satisfaction Report: Case Management Program

	The Miriam Hospital Score (National Mean)	
Category	August 1992	December 1993
Composite quality	94 (89)	90 (87)
Medical outcome	94 (87)	94 (88)
Physician care	96 (89)	93 (90)
Nursing care	94 (91)	93 (89)
Comfort/cleanliness	93 (83)	85 (84)
Food service	89 (76)	78 (77)
Admission/discharge	97 (87)	92 (88)
Other staff courtesy	96 (87)	88 (87)

Source: The Miriam Hospital. Used with permission.

Truly Integrated Systems

During 1994, the Miriam Hospital again faced mounting pressures from an unpredictable health care environment. Its case-mix index continues to rise while occupancy rates and LOS fluctuated during the first two quarters of the year. These occurrences, plus the potential for two new health plans in Rhode Island, have brought great pressure on the hospital to intensify its efforts to streamline delivery of care.

During these increasingly competitive times, the hospital will continue to expand its critical path/CareMap tool and case management systems. As a way to achieve full integration of the critical path/CareMap and case management programs, the clinical management team (composed of all clinical service chiefs, the vice-president of patient care services, the COO, and the CEO) will assume the steering committee function for both programs. This committee will be responsible for establishing and evaluating annual program goals, incorporating program goals into a hoshin plan for organization, and reviewing all appropriate related issues. Additionally, a staff physician has assumed a liaison position for these programs to the medical staff and will be responsible for increasing physician knowledge and participation. The Miriam Hospital also has adopted a formalized CQI process to address clinical issues that cannot be solved at the caregiver level. (See figure 3-18.) Examples of issues handled in this way might be the overall admitting or discharge planning process, or outpatient department hours and testing times. (See figure 3-14, p. 83.)

To date, the critical path/CareMap tool and case management systems have proven to be effective in meeting the changing requirements of patient care management at the Miriam Hospital. A future test for these programs will be the hospital's attainment of its strategic goal of becoming Rhode Island's highest-valued health care provider.

Case Example 3. The Medical Center

Montclair Baptist Medical Center (MBMC), located in Birmingham, Alabama, is a 534-licensed-bed hospital with 1993 admissions totaling 17,154 and an average LOS of 5.84 days. Its collaborative care model began in 1989 when the center was given a planning grant from the Robert Wood Johnson/PEW Charitable Trust's Strengthening Hospital Nursing. It had become clear to MBMC that if nursing were strengthened, everyone's roles and functions would be strengthened. However, it also became clear that everyone had to be involved in planning the changes in the overall patient care delivery system.

Figure 3-18. Clinical Improvement Team/High-Level Flow

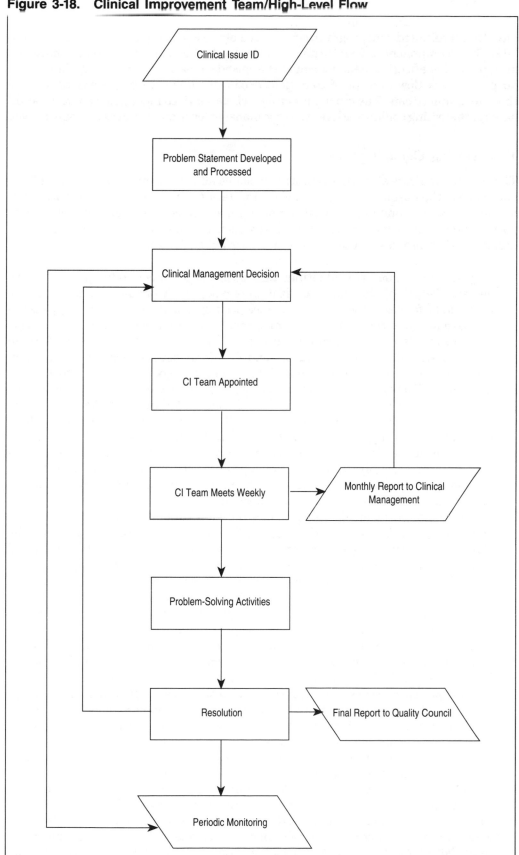

Source: The Miriam Hospital. Used with permission.

MBMC used a thoughtful combination of financial information (provided by Transition Systems Inc.), CQI processes, and *both* CareMap and case management strategies. Its coordinated care program is composed of the key components shown in figure 3-19. Those components currently unite at three levels to meet their organizational goals of (1) providing effective management of the episode of patient care, (2) redesigning the hospital's work flow to respond to patient needs, and (3) developing services to meet the continuum of care. The crucial junctures where services meet goals are the coordinated care steering committee level, the case manager level, and the direct caregiver level.

The Steering Committee Level

The coordinated care steering committee includes all key administrators (figure 3-20) and is one of the hospital's four principal committees. Given each year's changing external pressures, the committee's most important decision is that of determining target patient populations for formal collaborative care mechanisms. Clements and Love described that process in their article in *The New Definition*:

> The Steering Committee identifies target case types based on opportunities to decrease length of stay and/or utilization of resources. Consumer demands in the community for case type contractual price packaging also influence case type selection. An administrative project team is then formed for each selected case type.
>
> The administrative project team is chaired by a physician specialist in the clinical area who directs data analysis and CareMap development. The physician specialist is selected due to expressed interest in the project or by committee recommendation. They [the physician specialist] in turn develop a strategy to involve other physicians to strive toward the best demonstrated practice. Frequently, physicians from other specialties serve on the Task Force as well, i.e., Internal Medicine, Anesthesiology, Radiology, Pathology, etc. Other members of the Task Force include administrators, department heads, the nurse case manager, project director and financial analyst. Organizational processes to implement the best demonstrated practice for care of case type patients are evaluated and changes implemented for continuous improvement of quality.
>
> The Department of Finance provides decision support to determine the best demonstrated practice. Once the Steering Committee targets a new case type, the Clinical Cost Analyst performs an initial analysis of case type data. The initial analysis assists in delineation of the case type into a homogeneous group. This is accomplished through the use of a clinical assessment system that is part of the mainframe cost accounting system. The initial analysis of data begins with examination of the DRG to determine principal procedures and principal diagnoses within the DRG. Length of stay for principal diagnoses and procedures is determined as well as comorbidities and payor mix for the DRG. A detailed report of selected variables is run by medical department(s) and/or individual physician(s). The selected variables most often include: (1) variable cost per case, (2) daily nursing cost per case, (3) ancillary departmental cost per case, (4) average patient age, and (5) arithmetic and geometric average length of stay. For some case types, it is important for the project team to evaluate admit source for the patients as well as discharge disposition. The initial data plays a key role in determining clinically homogeneous patient groups within a DRG which can be defined into a case type.
>
> The initial analysis is presented to the case type project team. The finance department routinely receives requests from the project team to investigate practice issues and define utilization patterns to support development of a CareMap tool. Frequently, clinicians request dollar amounts be assigned to use of resources. Therefore, decisions for improvement of care are made with clinical judgement and financial information at the project team's fingertips.

Figure 3-19. Coordinated Care Program Key Components

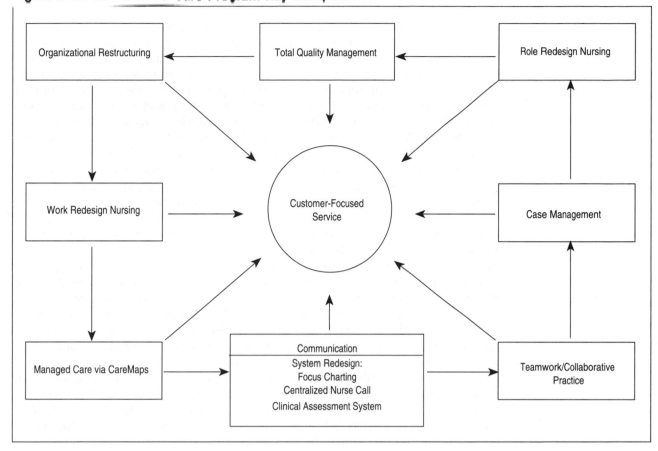

Figure 3-20. MBMC Coordinated Care Steering Committee

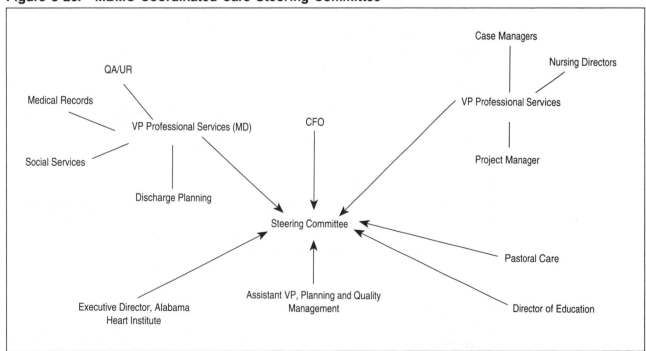

Source: MBMC. Used with permission.

Analysis requested by the team concerning use of resources may be as simple as a single lab test, radiology procedure or complex deciphering of an ICD-9 code rule. A table is developed to define variance in practice patterns. For example, Dr. Smith orders a CBC lab test on 80% of his cases and Dr. Jones orders only a hematocrit on 90% of her cases. A variable cost is calculated for the CBC and hematocrit. The physicians then determine whether cost/quality/service improvements are possible through change in routine practice patterns. Often the project team requires comparison of admissions by day of week and corresponding length of stay. This is useful in case types with a short length of stay to evaluate whether required testing/resources are readily available and/or expedient on weekends. Comparison of postoperative length of stay by surgeon with the day of stay that surgery occurred often shows unexpected opportunities for improvement. Information occasionally is needed from another regional or national data source. The Finance department is able to link with other systems to provide the comparative information needed.

Finance has the ability to analyze almost any financial or clinical situation that is needed to speed the development of the CareMap tool. The nurse case manager, in collaboration with the Administrative Project Team, organizes an interdisciplinary–interdepartmental team of caregivers to develop a CareMap tool. The CareMap document outlines patient needs, intermediate patient goals, and desired patient outcomes for the anticipated length of stay. Tasks and activities for care of the patient are outlined for each day of the anticipated length of stay. A version of the CareMap tool is developed for patients/families to increase their understanding of and participation in the episode of care.

Analysis of controllable cost per discharge for FY 91/92 revealed a total cost savings of $679,673.00 for the ten targeted case types. An additional ten case types were targeted for FY 92/93 and will be evaluated in July 93. Achievement of objectives related to the 20 case types by June 31, 1993, will result in 45% of inpatients at Montclair being managed by this process.

The financial impact of the program is also reflected in analysis of organizational operating expense as percentage of net revenue. The table below reflects accomplishments in this area:

Year	Percent
1991	89.5%
1992	86.0%
1993	79.5%

Implementation costs for FY 90/91 and FY 91/92 are estimated to be $490,000 with analysis for FY 92/93 due in July, 1993. This figure includes salary expense for the project director and nurse case managers.[9]

The Case Manager Level

There are 11 case managers who are not part of staffing assigned to 11 specialty areas. These are:

1. Cardiovascular (medical and surgical)
2. Pulmonary
3. Medicine
4. Diabetes
5. Orthopedics
6. Oncology
7. Neurology
8. OB/GYN

9. Neonatology
10. Surgery
11. Psychiatry

The case managers work Monday through Friday and expedite care through the various care areas. Because they facilitated collaborative development of the CareMap tools, they know the details and expert personnel intimately and thus can readily anticipate care as well as problem-solve specific individual patient situations.

Once the case managers are oriented to the acute phase of their assigned specialty's care, they begin to expand the scope of the program to care before and after the acute phase. At times, there has been overlap between case managers, discharge planners, utilization review, and preadmissions service nurses, which currently is being reviewed.

The case managers integrate the work of all disciplines by maintaining a focus on intermediate goals and outcomes. At present, they are formally accountable for the financial outcomes detailed on the CareMap tool. Within nursing, MBMC is redesigning nursing care delivery systems at the unit level to move accountability for the outcomes of nursing care to designated bedside staff nurses. As this important designation of accountability occurs, the case managers will be able to do several important things, including:

- Case-manage care across wider episodes including home care and prevention
- Zero in and spend more time with the catastrophic, complex case types and their multidisciplinary teams
- Incorporate other functions in the case manager role, such as discharge planning

The Direct Caregiver Level

The direct caregivers of each discipline refer to the CareMap tool. In 1991, the Medical Records Committee approved the CareMap form for use in the permanent record, whereas the medical department approves the content of each map. Using the CareMap only as a guide and not documentation had proven ineffective.

At this time, CareMap tools provide a multidisciplinary care plan and set up a system for charting by exception in progress notes; that is, the variances are the exception. (The case managers review the progress notes to collect data on all variances for analysis and reporting through hospital QA/QI channels.) Eventually, the amount of variances will be decreased to those that the collaborative groups believe to be crucial to increased costs, LOS, or poor clinical outcomes.

At this time, physicians and nonnursing disciplines do not document on the CareMap tools. Eventually, MBMC will move to this full function use on paper or upon purchasing an automated medical record system.

A major strength of the MBMC program is its comprehensive evaluation. Evaluation should be designed at the same time the program is designed. MBMC calls its evaluation a blueprint, and continues to review and revise it yearly. As figure 3-21 shows, MBMC's evaluation areas include patient satisfaction, physician satisfaction, nursing perception of quality, RN job satisfaction, controllable cost per discharge, and implementation costs.

Conclusion

A number of steps are involved in translating a collaborative care concept into a working program that will enable a health care organization to achieve the goal of lowering the cost of care without sacrificing the quality of care. Initially, the program must meet four criteria: (1) It must set annual overall and case-specific goals that can be

Figure 3-21. Coordinated Care Program Evaluation Budget

Objective	Method	Sample	Data Collection
	Coordinated Care Program Evaluation Blueprint FY 94 Montclair Baptist Medical Center		
Improve patient satisfaction	• Concurrent rounds	All nursing units	Ongoing
	• Written survey on day of discharge		
	• Telephone survey of patients two weeks post discharge		
Improve physician satisfaction	• Survey adapted from marketing tool	7th floor—5 to 10 physicians with high volume	Pre-October 1993 Post-May 1994
	• Corporate marketing tool	All nursing units	Biannually
Improve nurse satisfaction	• Index work satisfaction	7th floor RNs	Pre-September 1993
	• Nurse's perception of quality		Post-May 1994
Quality of care	• Average nurse response time	All nursing units	Ongoing
	• CareMap variance report	All targeted case types	Ongoing
	• Financial variance report	All targeted case types	Ongoing
Decrease cost per discharge	• Cost accounting system	All targeted case types	Quarterly

Source: Montclair Baptist Medical Center, Birmingham, AL. Used with permission.

quantitatively and qualitatively evaluated on a regular basis; (2) the program's goals must be doable within the facility's region and sociopolitical environment; (3) a direct relationship must exist between the program's goals and the processes and structures designed to achieve them; and (4) the people working on the collaborative care model must be given the authority and new-skill education to fulfill their responsibilities.

Once these criteria have been met, the organization, if it is truly serious about establishing a collaborative care program, must build a well-defined infrastructure that will guide program implementation and evaluation. Typically, this infrastructure will include a steering committee from the executive level, a full-time collaborative care program manager, and self-managing teams that will be active in authoring collaborative care techniques. The heart of collaborative care, these teams generally are of three types: direct-care teams, patient population (case type) teams, and program-level teams.

The value of the diversity of collaborative care programs currently in existence is that they can be customized to meet the needs of different organizations. This chapter has presented case studies demonstrating how three different organizations—a regional hospital, a community teaching hospital, and a medical center—have modified basic collaborative care principles to fit their individual needs. The case studies also show how they used different evaluation techniques to determine the success of their programs.

References

1. Henry, S. Conference proceedings from Case Management: Operationalizing Health Reform, Tucson, Apr. 25, 1994. Sponsored by Carondelet St. Mary's, Carondelet St. Joseph's, and CCM.

2. Griffin, D. Collaborative Case Project. Newton, MA: Newton-Wellesley Hospital, 1991.

3. Lumsdon, K. The AHA NOVA Awards: making collaboration work. *Hospitals and Health Networks* 68(2):42, Jan. 20, 1994.

4. DeHart, K. A report of the medical staff. In: *LRGH 1993 Annual Report.* Laconia, NH: LRGH, 1994, p. 4.

5. Lumsdon, K. Beyond four walls. *Hospitals and Health Networks* 68(5):45, Mar. 5, 1994.

6. Lipman, H., 1994. *LRGH 1993 Annual Report.* Used with permission.

7. Lumsdon, The AHA NOVA Awards, p. 44.

8. Walton, M. *The Deming Management Method.* New York City: Dodd, Mead & Co., 1986, pp. 86–88.

9. Clements, F., and Love, K. Decision support for coordinated care financial and clinical integration. *The New Definition* 8(4):1–3, Fall 1993.

CHAPTER FOUR

CareMap Project Management

Susan P. Kyzer

Once a collaborative care project has been designed and an infrastructure created to guide its implementation, it is ready to be transformed from concept into reality. The individual who is key to that transformation is the project manager. It is in effect the project manager, appointed by the executive steering committee, who has overall responsibility for coordinating the planning, implementation, and evaluation of the project. He or she must work with representatives from all levels of the organization to develop a system that everyone involved in the process can support and that will succeed in helping the organization reach its goals.

This chapter describes the phases of a CareMap project, identifies the key goals to be achieved at each phase, and outlines the education needed to prepare staff for project implementation. It also focuses on the role of the project manager and identifies common obstacles to avoid in the process of implementing a CareMap system.

The Project Phases

As discussed in chapter 1, a CareMap tool can be used to build and conduct collaborative care. It began as an expansion of the clinical path concept to include clinical progressions estimated against a planned time frame of care. Called intermediate goals and outcomes, these progressions constitute ongoing patient/family evaluation criteria.

The CareMap project proceeds in five phases. These phases provide a functional approach in that specific objectives can be assigned to each and the phases are chronological in nature. The five phases are:

1. Assessment and planning
2. Design
3. Pilot
4. Implementation
5. Evaluation and integration

Figure 4-1 gives an overview of phase objectives, the steps to obtain them, and the educational components involved in the development of a CareMap system.

Figure 4-1. Project Management: CareMap Project Phases

Phases and Objectives	Steps	Education
Phase 1: Assessment and Planning To provide infrastructure, resources, and direction for the project To provide a framework for future evaluation of the project	1. Appoint a steering committee. 2. Define administrative support. 3. Appoint a project manager. 4. Define roles. 5. Identify problems and issues. 6. Gather information. 7. Set goals. 8. Identify evaluation parameters and collect baseline data.	Provide information and expert resources to steering committee and medical staff regarding CareMaps, their purpose, benefits, and expected results.
Phase 2: Design To identify case types for pilot To develop content for CareMaps useful to clinicians in coordination of patient care To design forms that support the project goals To develop plans for education and monitoring to facilitate orderly and consistent implementation	1. Select 1 to 5 case types for pilot. 2. Identify content writing teams. 3. Appoint a task force to develop the format for the CareMaps and variance record and their guidelines. 4. Establish a process for monitoring implementation of the new tools. 5. Develop an education plan.	Provide information to all clinical departments regarding the CareMap project, including: • Basic terms • Goals of project • Writing teams • Task forces
Phase 3: Pilot To discover ways to improve the forms, content, and written guidelines and make revisions prior to general implementation To ascertain that variance data being recorded are useful	1. Combine content and format to produce a draft of the CareMap and variance record. 2. Pilot CareMaps on 5 to 10 patients within the selected case types. 3. Revise forms, content, and guidelines as many times as needed to arrive at a workable model.	Provide information for staff involved in the pilot regarding roles and responsibilities specific to the department or position, including: • Purpose of tools • How to use tools • How to manage variance
Phase 4: Implementation To provide clinicians with a CareMap tool to coordinate patient care, engage in collaborative practice, and manage care toward patient outcomes with efficient use of resources To collect clinical information useful for guiding care concurrently and determining trends and patterns that can be addressed through quality improvement processes	1. Implement CareMaps on all patients within the selected case types. 2. Monitor implementation process and address issues regarding the tools and system and accountability. 3. Identify appropriate channels for variance data and establish flow of reports.	Repeat education for additional groups of clinicians and support staff prior to implementation of CareMaps on their units. Provide ongoing support and continue to educate staff toward collaborative, outcome-based practice. Provide ongoing support and continue to educate staff toward recording and acting on variance concurrently.
Phase 5: Evaluation and Integration To evaluate progress toward identified goals To move from a project status to a fully integrated system that achieves and maintains the identified goals of the institution	1. Evaluate the project. 2. Incorporate CareMap tools into the medical record and streamline documentation where possible. 3. Integrate variance data into the QA/QI systems. 4. Include behaviors that support the use of CareMaps and variance management into performance appraisals.	Reinforce education as needed about specific issues that are problematic or as requested by staff. Continue to build skills needed for outcome-based, collaborative practice.

Phase 1. Assessment and Planning

This phase often begins as the result of a strategic planning process initiated by an organization in an effort to respond to pressures brought by outside sources, such as the community or the federal government. During this phase, the identification of objectives – for example, to document patient and family outcomes, to reduce length of stay (LOS), or to maintain or improve quality of care – leads administrators to focus on pragmatic solutions such as case management and CareMap systems. The ability of such clinical systems to achieve both cost and quality outcomes has been well documented in the literature.[1-4]

Objectives and Implementation

The assessment and planning phase has two immediate objectives: (1) to provide infrastructure, resources, and direction for the project; and (2) to provide a framework for future evaluation of the project. Achievement of these objectives is realized through implementation of the following sequence of steps.

Step 1. Appoint the Steering Committee

The steering committee is a key element in the infrastructure required to start the CareMap project. Because it is a decision-making body, its membership should include individuals who have the authority to make necessary changes. The committee should be multidisciplinary with member representatives from all involved departments. The core of the committee consists of a group of department heads from all the clinical departments (including the medical staff), utilization review (UR), quality assurance (QA), medical records, and information services. This group can be fairly large because it is a forum for information sharing and decision making.

The committee's overall function is to provide leadership for the collaborative care program. It oversees the implementation process and continually evaluates the program's design and function in light of the organization's mission. (See chapter 3 for a complete discussion of steering committee responsibilities.) Generally, the steering committee will need to meet monthly for at least the first year of the project.

Step 2. Define Administrative Support

Defining the type and amount of support that can be given to this project is the first step in planning. Resources that are needed include time from personnel at the executive, management, and staff levels to participate in development of the system, appointment of a full-time project manager, secretarial support for the project, information services support, supplies, and printing capabilities.

Step 3. Appoint the Project Manager

If possible, the project manager position should be full-time. The project's success will depend in large part on having someone who can devote as much time as possible to the development of the numerous facets of the CareMap system. If a full-time position is out of the question, the individual filling the role of project manager should be someone whose regular responsibilities are extremely flexible and would enable him or her to divide time appropriately between the two functions. The project manager's function and responsibilities are detailed in the next section of this chapter.

Step 4. Define Roles, Purpose, Accountabilities, Goals, and Educational Needs of Each Department

The steering committee's next step is to clearly define the roles, purpose, and accountabilities of each department. Special attention should be given to defining the impact of the CareMap system on areas such as utilization review/management, quality assurance/management, and discharge planning. Duplication of activities can be avoided in this way and planning for future integration of systems can begin. Additionally, every department needs to identify its own particular goals or hopes for the project and the educational needs of its members. For example, the social work department may have a goal to see certain kinds of patients soon after admission instead of being notified immediately prior to discharge.

Step 5. Identify Current Problems and Issues
Identifying current problems, issues, or concerns often helps to shape project goals. For example, a hospitalwide issue might be to successfully compete for managed care contracts, resulting in a goal to reduce the cost per case while maintaining high-quality outcomes. A department level concern might be the amount of time clinicians spend documenting, resulting in a goal to streamline documentation.

Step 6. Gather Information and Clarify Concepts
This step precedes goal setting. Once problems and issues have been identified, the information gathered about them can help clarify concepts that will begin to shape the project's goals. For example, past performance data such as LOS and cost per case may reveal opportunities for improvement. Likewise, information about physician practice patterns, when available, will show the degree of variation in current practice and may suggest how that variation affects outcomes. Present trends in data and future desires, based in part on available benchmark data, also prepare for the next step of setting goals. For example, if regional or national data are available regarding LOS for a certain diagnosis-related group (DRG) and a hospital's LOS is above the average, a future goal might be to reduce the LOS.

Step 7. Set Clear, Measurable Goals
Setting clear, measurable goals is extremely important to project success. Well-defined goals will give the project direction, and measurable goals will enable the results of the project to be evaluated. Goals should be concrete and realistic, and should focus on the most important four or five reasons for pursuing the project. Short-term or intermediate goals (such as having a certain number of CareMaps implemented by a certain month) should always be subject to the achievement of long-term goals. For example, while writing a CareMap tool for an elective surgical procedure, the writing team might discover the need for a presurgical patient education program. Rather than write a map for the current procedure, it might be of greater long-term value to explore the presurgical patient education program and then design the CareMap to include it. If the changes that need to be made are too far-reaching to be accomplished within a suitable time frame, the map could be written and revised after the new program is in place.

Step 8. Identify Basic Evaluation Parameters and Collect Baseline Data
Once clear, measurable goals have been set, it will be possible to identify basic evaluation parameters. Collecting the appropriate baseline data will allow for accurate evaluation of project results. If the hospital has access to a statistician, that expertise should be used to design simple but valid processes for evaluation.[5] Areas often used for evaluation include financial data, LOS, variability in practice, patient/family satisfaction, and staff/physician satisfaction. It is frustrating to feel that progress has been made but cannot be demonstrated because comparable baseline data are not available.

Education

During the planning and assessment phase, the exposure of project participants to published literature will almost certainly return dividends. Numerous articles have

been written by various disciplines and published in a variety of journals.[6-10] Building consensus about the project is the educational goal at this phase, as well as attain-
ing a consistent understanding of the project's basic concepts. The steering committee
will need information on what CareMap and case management systems are, their various purposes and benefits, and the results that have been experienced by other, similar hospitals or institutions.[11-13] Additionally, this may be a good time to bring in a
consultant or other expert in collaborative care project management to speak to the
group or to send key persons to a workshop on project management and have them
report back to the group.

Phase 2. Design

The design phase of the project involves making a number of decisions that will determine the project's direction. To select members to serve on the various task forces,
the steering committee must decide which case types to include in the project, which
settings will be used (emergency department, intensive care unit, outpatient, and so
on), over what continuum care will be provided (preop testing, rehab, home service,
and so on), and what staffs will be involved.

Objectives and Implementation

The design phase has four essential objectives: (1) to identify case types (patient populations) for the pilot phase, (2) to develop content for the CareMaps that will be used
by clinicians in the coordination of care, (3) to design forms that support the project
goals, and (4) to develop education and evaluation plans for use in project implementation. Achievement of these goals is realized through implementation of the following sequence of steps.

Step 1. Select Case Types for the Pilot Phase

Based on information gathered during the assessment and planning phase, the steering committee selects between one and five case types for the pilot phase. Typical indicators for case type selection include a high volume of patients, a predictable pattern
of care, physician/staff interest, availability of a well-managed area for the pilot, and
an apparent opportunity for improvement.

Step 2. Identify Content Writing Teams for Selected Case Types

Once case types have been selected, a content writing team for each can be identified.
Direct caregivers with expertise in a particular case type are the team's core members. However, other persons may be invited to join the team for a particular purpose.
For example, someone from materials management might be invited by the total hip
replacement team to discuss the cost of hip implants. Each content writing team is
assisted by a physician expert who supplies the medical plan that forms the basis
for the CareMap development. The medical plan may be the current practice pattern
of that particular physician or the best-practice-pattern consensus of the physicians
who will be using the CareMap tool. The kind of CareMap tool the team writes will
depend on the situation that exists within the physician group that cares for that
specific case type. For example, physicians organized around service lines may already
have developed protocols, guidelines, or standing orders that outline what is, by their
consensus, a best-practice pattern. However, physicians who practice in isolation have
little way of comparing their practice methodology to that of their peers. In this
scenario, it will take longer for physicians to form a cohesive group and develop a best-
practice map. Regardless, it is important that everyone know that "best practice" is
the eventual goal even if current practice maps are being written first.

Step 3. Appoint a Task Force to Develop Formats for the CareMap Tool and the Variance Record and to Develop Guidelines for Their Use

At the same time that writing teams are developing the content of the CareMaps, another task force is developing their format. The format of the CareMap tool determines what it will look like and is designed to support the goals of the project. If the map is to become part of the medical record, it must be designed to meet medical record requirements (margin size, where patient information appears, and so on). Additionally, the format will vary according to the amount of documentation to be incorporated into the CareMap and which disciplines want to streamline their documentation processes. If the CareMap is a part of the medical record it can replace other forms such as the nursing care plan. When the CareMap combines or replaces care plans and additional forms, caregivers will welcome the opportunity to decrease time spent on paperwork. Documentation issues are discussed in further detail in chapter 7.

The method for recording variances also must be determined during this phase. As explained in chapter 1, *variances* are different or unexpected events or occurrences in the process of care delivery that serve to show where the CareMap plan differs from reality. (See chapter 6 for a complete discussion of variance.) The format for the variance record must be developed, and guidelines must be written for using both the CareMap tool and the variance record. The task force responsible for the variance record should include direct caregivers from each department who will be documenting in the CareMap. Representatives from medical records, QA, QI, UR, discharge planning, and information services also should be included.

Variance management issues are many and complex. The following questions illustrate some of the issues to be addressed:

- Who will record the variance?
- Who will collect and aggregate the data?
- How will the data be stored?
- Who will analyze the data?
- What kind of reports might be useful from the variance data?

A second phase of work for this task force might be to begin to explore integration of variance data into existing systems such as UR, QA, and continuous quality improvement (CQI).

Step 4. Establish a Process for Monitoring Implementation of the New Tools

A process for monitoring the pilot and implementation process must be established to ensure the orderly and consistent use of the CareMap tool. Those in direct supervisory positions should be made responsible for helping their employees learn the new behaviors required by a CareMap system. Specific behaviors should be delineated to managers and staff so that expectations are clear. The use of a simple audit tool with entries such as "CareMap complete," "signature present," "variance recorded as appropriate," and so on allows for peer review, self-review, and management review and helps monitor the process. A regular meeting of all managers to discuss problems with implementation, share successes, and provide peer support during the pilot and implementation of the CareMap tools will be of great help.

Step 5. Develop an Education Plan

A plan for educating all clinical staff about the CareMap system will make everyone involved feel informed and included in the project. The timing of the education offered depends on the progression of the project. The persons responsible for developing and implementing the education plan will vary with the institution, but should include the project manager and a representative from the education department. Whether the education department actually presents some of the education sessions or only serves as a support in setting up in-services depends in large part on its internal resources and structure. In either case, the project manager will be instrumental in developing the content of the presentations and will play a major role in the education process. Others who may be involved formally (and certainly informally) are those who have 24-hour accountability for patient care, such as unit managers, assistant managers, supervisors, and department directors.

Education

The initial education provided in this phase should include an overview of basic terms and concepts so that everyone begins with the same framework. Often terms in the literature are confusing and have different meanings in different articles. Providing a glossary of terms for the project would be a good way to promote consistency in the way terms are used within the institution. Presentation of the project goals will give caregivers a basis for understanding the purpose for the changes being made. Information on the various task forces and their responsibilities will be interesting to staff and will show them how they can participate in developing a system that will result in improved coordination of patient care.

Education for management staff should include methods for helping them cope with change.[14-16] Understanding change, identifying individual responses to change, and knowing what to expect from staff during projects requiring change in work behaviors is a necessary component of any manager's job in the current health care environment. Offering a workshop or a retreat where these issues can be formally addressed is one way to support the management staff as well as to provide them the opportunity to build the team skills needed for collaboration.

After the initial education regarding the CareMap system is completed, other concepts that should be introduced to staff include outcome-based practice and collaborative practice. The staff skills needed for a CareMap system include critical thinking, negotiation, inclusion (that is, including team members in the work rather than delegating work), and follow-up/follow-through.[17-21] The amount of education on these issues will depend in part on previous training and an assessment of current staff skill level and needs.

Other useful approaches to providing information on CareMap tools would be to set up presentations of basic concepts and project plans institutionwide, to offer in-services on outcome-based practice and collaborative practice, to put a CareMap system "update" on each department's or unit's agenda, and to either place articles on CareMaps in the institution's newsletter or create a special CareMap newsletter.

Phase 3. Pilot

The pilot phase allows a limited number of staff to be exposed to the new tool in a closely monitored and controlled situation. Working out the mechanics of how the tool will actually perform with staff who have been a part of the development process will improve the tool's chance for success. During this phase, staff will evaluate the CareMap tool for appropriate wording, ease of use, accuracy of content, clarity of guidelines, and so on. During this time, the project manager should be in close contact with staff on the various pilot units.

Objectives and Implementation

The pilot phase has two specific objectives: (1) to discover ways to improve the project's forms, content, and written guidelines and to make revisions prior to general implementation; and (2) to ascertain that the variance data being recorded are useful. Achievement of these objectives is realized through implementation of the following sequence of steps.

Step 1. Combine Content and Format to Produce a Draft of the CareMap Tool and the Variance Tracking Record

After the tasks in the design phase have been completed, the content of the CareMap developed by the writing team must be combined with the format chosen by the task force to produce a usable draft. This step requires an individual skilled in the use of word processing or forms software. A draft that can be produced using the copy machine will save time and money. Because rapid and frequent revisions are crucial during this phase, sending the CareMap to a printer is neither efficient nor cost-effective.

Step 2. Pilot CareMap(s) on 5 to 10 Patients

The draft document is used for the first 5 to 10 patients with the case type description who are admitted to the area piloting the CareMap tool. During this time, close monitoring of the tool occurs and staff members record and report any problems with its use. They also record variances and any problems encountered with wording, clarity, and so on. After the first pilot is completed, the responsible task forces discuss the results. Format issues are reviewed by each task force, and content and variance results are reviewed by the respective writing teams.

Step 3. Revise Forms, Content, and Written Guidelines as Often as Needed to Arrive at a Workable Tool

The various task forces then revise the forms, content, and guidelines according to feedback from the staffs using the new tools. After revising and using the draft tools with another 5 to 10 patients, the results are reviewed again. This loop is continued until the staff members in the pilot areas feel that CareMap and variance tracking tools have been developed that will work. The content writing team also should look at the variance data to determine if the desired information has been obtained. Every effort should be made to ensure that the variance information recorded is meaningful. For example, initially it is common for staff to attribute many variances to "lack of physician order" rather than considering the underlying reasons. If an IV is not discontinued, for example, the underlying reason might be that the patient suffered nausea or that the hematocrit was low and the line was needed for transfusion. Thus, in this scenario the lack of physician order is not the real cause of the variance. Staff will quickly learn what to record on the variance record if they are given feedback and reports about variance. Even at best, the tools will not be perfect and thus the pilot period should not be prolonged unreasonably. The objective is to achieve a tool that clinicians are able to use rather than "the perfect CareMap."

The project manager and the unit manager should be readily available during this time. Informal discussions of what the guidelines mean in certain situations, how to record specific variances, whether wording of the content is clear, and so on will give them insight into what the mechanical and logistical problems are with the forms and the system as designed. Many of the problems revolve around how terms and goals are defined and how information is communicated from shift to shift and department to department. No problem is trivial at this stage, and the project manager should be prepared to provide a lot of support and encouragement. One desired outcome of this phase is that staff will feel themselves to be an integral part of the process of solving problems they identify. Their perception that suggestions are acted on rapidly and result in the improvement of the CareMap tool will encourage further participation.

Education

After the CareMap tool(s), the variance tracking record, and operational guidelines are completed (but prior to their first "trial run"), the staff directly involved must receive detailed instruction about how to use the tools. This information should be department or unit specific and should be very concrete. The purpose of the tools, how to use them, and how to manage any variances should be discussed and practiced. The guidelines probably will need to be clarified at this point as staff have questions that are not addressed adequately. Practice situations where staff have the actual forms to write on and "try out" the new system are very important to their comfort level when the pilot period begins. Although the pilot area is limited, the education effort is great because all staff coming in contact with the CareMap must be educated. It is important to emphasize to staff that their honest feedback is crucial to the development of the CareMap tool as a workable document.

As the pilot phase begins, most of the formal education for the staff of the pilot unit(s) has been completed. Having resources available to staff to answer questions, reinforce new behavior, help problem-solve, and provide encouragement is extremely important. Having someone knowledgeable available to assist staff in using the new tools will be especially important on off-shifts and weekends. The first time a person tries any new behavior is a critical learning period, and it is important that that individual have as many positive experiences as possible.

A number of techniques may be used to make the learning process easier and more rewarding. These include providing department-, unit-, or shift-based in-service education; using self-instruction materials; and using mock patient chart exercises to practice filling out new forms.

Phase 4. Implementation

Implementation of the CareMap project is perhaps the most difficult phase because it involves a greater number of staff and thus more extensive education and monitoring. During this phase, the usual methods for maintaining staff accountability must begin to replace the almost one-on-one nurturing that the project manager provided the pilot staff. The now-workable CareMap tools can be implemented with all patients in the selected case types. As more case types are developed and more units or areas are involved, the education process is repeated. Once all staff have been educated in the use of the CareMap tool and the variance tracking record, implementation of other CareMaps is readily accomplished.

Objectives and Implementation

The implementation phase has two principal objectives: (1) to provide clinicians with a CareMap tool to coordinate patient care, engage in collaborative practice, and manage care toward patient outcomes with efficient use of resources; and (2) to collect clinical information useful for guiding care concurrently and determining trends and patterns that can be addressed through quality improvement processes. Achievement of these objectives is realized through implementation of the following sequence of steps:

Step 1. Implement CareMaps on All Patients within the Selected Case Types
Each admitted patient meeting the case type description is now placed on the appropriate CareMap. Admission procedures should be revised to reflect how this will be accomplished and who will be accountable for selecting the CareMap tool. Working as a team, all staff involved in the patient's care will now use the CareMap tool to help that patient reach the desired outcomes in a timely, cost-effective way. Variances to the CareMap will alert staff to take corrective action when possible.

Step 2. Monitor Implementation Process and Address Issues regarding the Tools, System, and Accountability
Managers from every department using and documenting on the CareMap will now monitor patient care according to the plan they developed. Clear guidelines of expected

behavioral changes and activities should be in place so that consistent direction can be given to staff members. The management team should continue to think about positive ways to educate and support the staff in this major change. Specific criteria should be used to audit utilization of the CareMap; inter-shift, intradisciplinary, and intradepartmental communication; and variance recording.

As the CareMap and variance tools are being implemented, close monitoring should occur to ensure that staff are using them, understand them, and have an opportunity to give feedback about the system. Any problems should be taken seriously and addressed as quickly as possible. Staff should be encouraged to speak up without fear of being labeled as "resistant to change." Every department should be held accountable for its own participation in the CareMap system, and it is important that no one department assume a "policing" role in which it tries to ensure that others follow through with their responsibilities.

As the project involves more staff, department and unit managers must become comfortable with monitoring the implementation process. Rather than perceiving the CareMap system as yet another thing to be "checked on," managers should view it as a tool that will greatly assist them in performing their basic job functions. Ultimately, managers are accountable for the care delivered within their area of responsibility and for the staff that delivers that care. CareMap tools make it easier to determine patient progress toward outcomes and give managers concrete information about which staff are delivering care in an organized fashion. Having this information enables managers to assist staff in improving care in a specific and constructive fashion. Honest, objective feedback to staff about their performance given in a positive supportive way will facilitate learning.

Step 3. Identify Appropriate Channels for Variance Data and Establish Flow of Reports

Once variance data are collected, they should be sent to the appropriate group to be analyzed and acted on.[22] The steering committee identifies which data are significant to which functions of the institution and determines the channels through which to send those data, apprising all involved staff (including the medical staff) of what will be done with the data. For example, variance data on patient education outcomes might be channeled to the nursing QA committee, data on ordering certain antibiotics might be channeled to the pharmacy and therapeutics committee, data on certain clinical complications might be sent to the medical QA committee, and data on the unavailability of a certain test on the weekends might be sent to a CQI team to investigate.

Education

The education related to the actual use of the CareMap tool and the variance record must be repeated for all groups of staff who will be using them. Staff should receive the ongoing support of management to develop the skills needed for outcome-based practice and collaborative practice. Continuing education on and reinforcement of concurrent variance management should be provided. Additionally, staff must be clear on their authority to act on variance information.

As the project progresses to the full implementation stage, additional education should be in response to specific needs identified by staff and management. As always, reinforcement and encouragement should be ongoing, and everyone should be kept informed of the project's progress. Successes should be advertised and should include day-to-day as well as major goal achievements. The hospital newsletter is a good forum for regular project updates and spotlights.

As with the previous phases, a number of techniques may be used to enhance and ensure the learning process. For example, managers should be provided with peer support structures to discuss any problems and their role in further developing staff, focus groups might be held from time to time to allow staff to give feedback about new tools and practice expectations, and positive behavior and success should be spotlighted and celebrated.

Phase 5. Evaluation and Integration

The final phase involves evaluating progress toward project goals and moving from project status to program integration into existing or restructured institutional systems. When the project becomes part of the existing systems, the project manager should be able to focus on developing additional CareMap content teams or further phases of project development, and the system should continue to function and maintain the objectives that have been achieved thus far.

Objectives and Implementation

The evaluation and integration phase has a number of objectives: (1) to evaluate progress toward goals, both the project's and the institution's; (2) to move from a project status to an integrated system having the support of administration; (3) to integrate the variance data into QA/QI systems; (4) to ensure that patient care is managed toward outcomes concurrently; and (5) to incorporate behaviors that support the system into job descriptions and performance appraisals at all levels. Achievement of these objectives is realized through implementation of the following sequence of steps.

Step 1. Evaluation

Evaluation of the goals of the project should occur almost constantly in order to keep the project on track. However, it is important to have formal evaluations provided in written reports at predetermined times – for example, at the end of each year of the project. Whatever criteria were set for evaluation at the beginning of the project are used to measure success. Sometimes an unexpected success can be included in the evaluation anecdotally even if no baseline data are available for comparison. Evaluation of goals will give guidance to the next steps to be taken. Learning from the experience of the first year, new goals can be set and a new plan formulated. Usually, integration of the CareMap system with mainline hospital systems is a gradual process.

Step 2. Incorporate CareMap Tools into the Medical Record and Streamline Documentation Where Possible

Accepting the CareMap tool as an integral part of the medical record is a pivotal point in integrating and maintaining the system. If the CareMap tool remains an additional piece of documentation and cannot take the place of other forms (such as the nursing care plan), it will be difficult to maintain staff enthusiasm. Consistent results can be achieved only with consistent use of the tools.

Step 3. Integrate Variance Data into QA/QI Systems

Program evaluation of cost and quality issues can be ongoing through analysis of variance data (both intervention and outcome), cost data, and patient/family satisfaction data.[23-29] Integration of appropriate variance data into existing systems such as QA/QI is important to avoid duplication of data collection. Issues discovered through the process of developing CareMaps or through variances can be addressed via the existing CQI process. For example, delay in obtaining electrocardiograms (EKGs) in the emergency department may show up as a pattern in variance recording. A CQI team might be formed to investigate this problem and recommend a plan of action to decrease waiting time for an EKG to be performed.

Step 4. Include Behaviors That Support Use of the CareMap
Tools and Variance Management in Job Descriptions
and Performance Appraisals

Accountability for patient outcomes should be determined within each department and clarified between various departments. How will these accountabilities be managed and monitored (for example, through performance appraisal)? What kind of care delivery system will be used (for example, primary nursing)? Will additional roles be utilized (for example, case manager)? What formal mechanisms for collaboration among disciplines will be established (for example, interdisciplinary rounds)? The answers to these questions will determine the way the system is integrated.

An overall assessment of the project's progress toward integration may address the seven characteristics of a fully integrated CareMap system outlined in figure 4-2. In addition to those issues, the presence of a goal related to the CareMap system or case management in the institution's strategic plan would indicate the executive team's commitment to the project. This commitment also would be reflected in the infrastructure set up to develop and support the project.

Another important issue is whether care is being planned and delivered for an episode of illness rather than for isolated segments of care. Have traditional boundaries been crossed to provide patients with continuity of care? Has the institution made it possible for formerly unrelated parts of the health care system to begin to collaborate to improve quality of service?

Operational restructuring may occur to reorganize processes to be multidisciplinary rather than department based. As roles within the institution and external requirements change, the executive staff must continually return to the basic questions: What work is to be done? and What is the best way to do it? Any restructuring should be in response to these questions and provide a better and not just a different way to do the work.

Education

Education for the evaluation and integration phase consists of reinforcing information as requested by staff for better utilization of the system or as indicated by problematic issues. Ongoing education regarding outcome-based practice and collaborative practice should be provided at intervals and incorporated into new-employee orientation. As mentioned earlier, skill building in areas such as critical thinking, negotiation, inclusion, and follow-up/follow-through must be long-term goals for staff development. Techniques that may be used to enhance this phase include reporting progress toward goals in the institution newsletter, sharing success stories, and providing formal evaluation reports at specified times and publicizing the results.

The Role of Project Manager

What is the work to be done? and Who will be responsible for doing it? are basic questions to any organization desiring or undergoing change. An efficient, effective way to make organizational change is, first, to define a project and, then, to appoint someone to be accountable for planning, developing, and implementing a plan designed to produce results. The phases of a CareMap project can be "mapped" out to provide the steering committee with a critical path to guide the process. Target dates can be set and strategies developed for each phase of the project. (See figure 4-3.) Managing these multifaceted processes and ensuring that everything fits together is part of the project manager's role. This role can be summarized in one short phrase: Make it happen! However, in order to make it happen, the project manager position must incorporate innumerable activities, responsibilities, and skills.

Figure 4-2. Characteristics of a Fully Integrated CareMap and/or Case Management System

	Not at all Haven't begun	Somewhat	Mostly	Fully
1. CareMap system and/or case management named specifically in institution's mission statement and year's goals?				
2. Infrastructure for CareMap system—Do you have:				
*Executive steering committee that meets at least quarterly?				
Full-time project manager?				
*Relationships clarified between CQI, UM, UR, QA, etc.?				
Regular review and feedback by collaborative clinician groups?				
Initial education of all staff and managers?				
*Comfort level and participation of department heads?				
Ongoing education of all staff and managers?				
3. CareMap as core of medical record				
*Legal issues resolved?				
Multidisciplinary in content?				
*Multidisciplinary in care management and variance recording?				
*Streamline permanent documentation?				
A patient/family version of CareMap tool?				
*Clarification of volume/type of variance data desired?				
4. Episodic-based care, beyond acute setting				
CareMaps describe care beyond traditional acute care boundaries where appropriate?				
People connected formally across boundaries?				
5. Accountability for outcomes formalized/clarified within each department				
*Nursing determines its infrastructure for case accountability?				
Physicians determine an infrastructure for continuity?				
Primary nursing?				
Case managers utilized?				
Collaborative practice group established?				
Other formal mechanisms?				
6. Program evaluation of cost/quality				
Variance data about interventions?				
*Variance data about outcomes				
*Data about cost, not charge per case?				
Research?				
Patient/family satisfaction data?				
7. Operational restructuring				

* = Critical challenges

Reprinted, with permission, from The Center for Case Management, Inc., South Natick, MA. Copyright 1993.

Job Description

Typically, the project manager job description is broad in order to allow full development of the role. Following are some of the areas that may be included:

- Responsibility for the development, implementation, and coordination of CareMap tools
- Responsibility for staff and patient/family education as related to the project
- Development of a system for management of variance data
- Facilitation of care coordination within the multidisciplinary team and between the multidisciplinary team and the medical staff
- Participation in institutionwide committees and professional development

Figure 4-4 provides a more comprehensive example list of project manager role functions.

Authority Base

The project manager's authority base should come from the highest, operational decision-making body. Because the project is institutionwide, authority also must be institutionwide. The project manager should have access to information and resources from every department. Having this privilege enables him or her to begin to understand how systems fit together and what each department's concerns and issues are

Figure 4-3.   Project Management: Sample Time Line

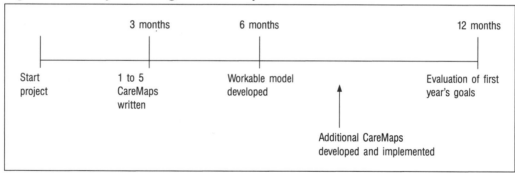

Figure 4-4.   Project Management: Sample Project Manager Role Functions

1. Develops a strategic plan for project with guidance from steering committee.
2. Implements and oversees strategic plan for project.
3. Assures ongoing CareMap development for selected patient populations.
4. Coordinates implementation of CareMaps.
5. Assists with orientation of staff to CareMap system.
6. Assists with development of teaching tools in relation to CareMaps.
7. Develops a plan for storage, retrieval, and use of variance data.
8. Facilitates system changes by referral or action plan.
9. Coordinates and is a liaison for all project task forces, groups, and committees.
10. Facilitates communication within multidisciplinary team.
11. Facilitates communication between medical staff and multidisciplinary team.
12. Participates on hospital and department committees.

in relation to the care of the selected patient populations. This knowledge will strengthen the project manager's role as coordinator, facilitator, and integrator of systems and as liaison between departments, disciplines, and people.

Personal Qualities

The project manager has to provide both leadership and labor for the project. The role contains a unique juxtaposition of philosophy and mechanics. For example, at a given moment the issue may be a discussion on how to define a patient outcome in language common to all disciplines and at the next it may be a discussion on the best place to fit the addressograph on the form.

The personal qualities of a successful project manager can be summarized by six key concepts. These are:

1. *Credibility:* This is the cornerstone of success for the project manager. Without it, it would be impossible to lead people to do new things. He or she must have credibility with physicians, administration, managers, and staff alike, which is a reason that often more rapid progress is possible at first when the project manager role is filled from within the organization. "Credibility, like reputation, is something that is earned over time. It does not come automatically with the job or the title."[30] A project manager brought in from outside will need extra time to build credibility, learn the culture and internal systems, and become an integral part of the organization.

2. *Flexibility:* This allows the project manager to generate a true sense of teamwork within the various groups and task forces that are working. There are many ways to do the same thing, and flexibility is needed so that different options can be explored. Looking beyond structure and detail to purpose and function sometimes can open the way to make truly innovative changes.

3. *Dependability:* Although this may be considered a subconcept of credibility, it deserves special emphasis. Doing what one says one will do when one says one will do it, and consistently, often is very difficult. In a situation where change is occurring rapidly and staff are being asked to participate in revising change as it happens, project manager dependability is crucial. Care should be taken to promise only what is truly possible (for example, promising that a revised form will come out by the end of the month).

4. *Problem-solving ability:* This is needed for thinking through both the conceptual issues that accompany major change and the detail-oriented problems of tool and system design. Problem-solving skills also are needed to help effect the system changes that need to occur. Having an institutionwide view of how systems affect patient care in specific ways gives the project manager a unique and powerful opportunity to help various parts of the organization become aware of and problem-solve these issues.

5. *Creativity:* In the project manager function, creativity can be "the spoonful of sugar that makes the medicine go down!" Although collaborative care project implementation is a complex and serious task, it should be made as pleasant and engaging as possible. The individual who tries to make the activities of the project interesting and creative will have more success throughout the process. From the first education sessions to the task force meetings to promotional "gimmicks" for the project, the project manager should add some special creative flair to pique interest and generate enthusiasm. For example, special table decorations in the cafeteria during the first week of implementation, buttons for team members, a contest to name the CareMap system, and posters and bulletin boards are some ideas that project managers have used with great success.

6. *Good interpersonal skills:* Possession of good interpersonal skills underlies all the other qualities that have been mentioned. The ability to communicate ideas to others and help them see value in doing things a different way is one of the project manager's main functions. The concept of leadership as a relationship, "... one characterized by serving others, rather than being served ..." is very valuable to the role of project manager.[31] He or she is involved in leading others to a better way of managing patient care and doing whatever tasks are necessary to enable others to participate in "making it happen."

Working Relationships

The project manager has to build a solid working relationship with three particular groups within the institution: the steering committee, the department directors, and middle management. Each of these groups looks to the project manager for a special kind of assistance.

The steering committee depends on the project manager to keep the project on track and to let the committee know if it needs to intervene to facilitate progress. The project manager must bring the committee all the information it needs to make appropriate decisions. In turn, each committee meeting's agenda should be clear so that the project manager knows what is needed to move the project along. Part of the project manager's role is to do as much foundational thinking, preparation, and negotiating as possible before committee meetings so that maximal progress can be attained. For example, to save time and minimize conflict, he or she should ensure that sensitive or controversial issues are addressed privately or in small groups before being brought to a full committee meeting for discussion.

Department directors depend on the project manager to help coordinate and execute much of the policy and procedure revision required by the new system. Because department directors are concerned principally with how the project is going to affect their procedures, budget, staffing, and accreditation issues, they will rely on the project manager's knowledge to help them make the adjustment. Thus, the project manager will facilitate the department directors' understanding of the project and promote realistic expectations of the new system.

Middle management depends on the project manager to help people bridge the gap between the project as a concept and the project as an integrated system. Because middle managers are primarily concerned with how the new system is going to affect the day-to-day operation of their area or unit, they need to know who is going to be responsible for what and how they are expected to make sure the work gets done. Additionally, middle managers need to know how their staff will be expected to communicate within and outside their area or unit. The project manager's support and facilitation expertise is particularly important with this group because it is at this level that the project will eventually succeed or fail.

From the first presentation of the project's basic concepts and goals, the project manager (as well as the steering committee) must attempt to engage the interest and enthusiasm of staff to participate. Gaining staff support of and commitment to the CareMap system is crucial to its success. Thus, the project manager must seek out and involve key players from every possible area, unit, discipline, and department of the organization who will be helpful and willing to talk openly about how things work from their perspective. These "champions" will help the project manager discover project attributes that will appeal to or meet a need of their particular area. When staff in that area are able to perceive the benefits offered by the new system, they will more readily embrace it.

Ideally, the champions are individuals who are found in areas or disciplines where there already is a lot of involvement with the project and who share the vision of what a CareMap system can do for patient care management. Because they are already participating in the process and recognize its value, they are extremely effective in helping those with whom they work to understand it and its desired result. Their enthusiasm contributes to a positive work environment. Often these champions are clinicians who have been involved on task forces, have volunteered to try the first CareMap tool, or have otherwise shown interest in going a little beyond what is normally expected. Typically, their interest has been cultivated through one-on-one relationships with the project manager or members of the steering committee in the course of their participation in informal discussions or on task forces and committees.

It is important to find champions at all levels and on all shifts. These are the people who will tell the project manager not only that something is not working, but why. The more champions a project manager has, the easier it will be to keep the project's momentum going.

Common Obstacles to Project Implementation

Numerous obstacles can slow the project's progress or even stop it for a time. These obstacles include limited vision and lack of commitment, lack of multidisciplinary involvement, documentation issues, concerns about variance data, lack of physician involvement, and legal issues. Some obstacles can be avoided or at least prepared for in an effort to avert major roadblocks.

Limited Vision and Lack of Commitment

Limited vision as to what a CareMap system can accomplish and lack of commitment on the part of the executive team often go together. It is important that the project not be perceived as a quick fix. This obstacle can be avoided by ensuring that everyone involved understands the project's significance and goals and that commitment to the project as a long-term, real improvement exists at the executive level. Information from literature and seminars or conferences can be shared; presentations by persons experienced with CareMap systems and informal and formal discussion can promote commitment to the project. Having the establishment of a CareMap system as a part of the institution's yearly goals indicates the level of commitment conducive to success. A fallout of lack of commitment is an inadequate allocation of resources to the project. Appointment of a full-time project manager will help ensure that the resources required to manage the project are clearly defined.

Lack of Multidisciplinary Involvement

Another common obstacle is that of trying to develop and implement the project out of any one department. For example, sometimes a CareMap project begins in the finance department as a measure to reduce costs, in the nursing department as a way to better coordinate care, or in the quality assurance department as a way to collect clinical data. It is important to include in the development of the system all the departments that will be involved in the implementation of the system. An executive-level steering committee will ensure that decisions are made in the best interests of the institution and help avoid turf issues that might arise between departments.

Documentation Issues

Documentation issues are real. Caregivers are not really interested in another piece of paper to handle and another place to chart. CareMap tools are much more appealing if they can replace other forms of documentation. Avoiding this obstacle can be time-consuming because it involves reviewing and revising the documentation system to streamline and integrate forms. Making the CareMap tool a part of the medical record at some point is the only way to decrease documentation. Although a large task, this usually is an area where clinicians are ready and willing to help. The rewards of this particular endeavor can be quite spectacular.

Concerns about Variance Data

Sometimes the organization's comfort level with the integration of variance data into the QA/QI systems can be an obstacle. One way to overcome it is to create clear guidelines about (1) what information will be collected, (2) to what persons or committees the information will flow, (3) what will be confidential and what will be made public, and (4) what statistics are reported and to whom. For example, LOS statistics might be reported but without physician names attached. Cost per case might be reported privately to physicians to allow them to compare their own practice to that of their peers. Information regarding frequency of complications could be dealt with through the medical staff QA mechanism to provide regular review-and-educate cycles.

Using variance data in any way that could possibly be construed as punitive is guaranteed to have a negative impact. This can be avoided by simply not doing it. Instead, it is important to stress the positive aspects of variance data reporting. For example, physicians may find it helpful to know the frequency of certain postsurgical complications experienced by patients. Physical therapists may find it useful to know (or want data to support) that earlier intervention results in earlier achievement of outcomes. Nurses may be interested in knowing how often patients must be recatheterized after removal of an indwelling catheter or whether teaching efforts are resulting in adequate patient knowledge. Prior to the CareMap system, this kind of clinical information could be obtained only by laborious chart review or conducting numerous "studies."

Lack of Physician Involvement

One way to avoid the obstacle of lack of physician involvement is to involve physicians in the project early on. Education about the project should be provided in the way most acceptable to each physician. For example, some may prefer to be informed via written material whereas others may prefer a brief explanation from the project manager or writing team leader. Presenting brief updates at medical staff meetings also is an effective way to involve many physicians. Other strategies include bringing in a speaker to address a physician group or sending one or more of the institution's leading physicians to workshops.

Legal Issues

Another obstacle to be addressed is that of the legal issues that often concern physicians. Physicians are rightfully concerned about maintaining control over their practice. By providing a way for them to be proactive in determining how the best-practice pattern is defined in the institution, the CareMap system returns that control to the physician group. Physicians are primarily concerned about the effect that the use of a CareMap might have on the incidence and outcome of malpractice litigation. From an examination of this issue, Nolin and Lang state, "Maps will probably tend to protect diligent providers while creating additional risk for careless providers, thus tending to place the incidence and outcome of liability suits on a more rational basis."[32] If other specific issues are troubling physicians, legal counsel should be sought from a knowledgeable source. No matter what anyone else says, physicians will want to hear from or read the perspective of a lawyer.

Conclusion

Project management is one of the most challenging roles facing the health care professional. Although demanding, it also is exciting and rewarding. The opportunity to participate in structuring new systems for patient-centered care is uniquely available in this time of unprecedented change. Project management is central to the successful development and implementation of CareMap and case management systems. The organization and orchestration of the project will determine how staff view it, how well they understand their participation in it, how effectively people and ideas are incorporated into the work, and eventually how successful the results are. CareMap and case management systems can play a vital part in reaching goals related to balancing cost and quality, and the project manager is one key to the successful implementation of these systems.

References

1. Flynn, A., and Kilgallen, M. Case management: a multidisciplinary approach to the evaluation of cost and quality standards. *Journal of Nursing Care Quality* 8(1):58-66, Oct. 1993.

2. Southwick, K. Two approaches to better outcomes at lower cost. *Strategies for Healthcare Excellence* 7(3):1-7, Mar. 1994.

3. Andersson, S. ScrippsHealth: quality planning for clinical processes of care. *The Quality Letter for Healthcare Leaders* 5(8):2-4, June 1993.

4. Hopkins, J., editor. Bridgeport Hospital: evolution revolutionizes climate for quality. *ORC Advisor* 9(5):1-6, 1993.

5. Weilitz, P., and Potter, P. A managed care system: financial and clinical evaluation. *The Journal of Nursing Administration* 23(11):51-57, Nov. 1993.

6. The next wave of hospital case management: mapping out psychiatric diagnoses on paths. *Hospital Case Management* 1(10):173-76, Oct. 1993.

7. Kleinman, J. Case management tool reduces length of stay, costs. *Innovations '92: The American College of Physician Executives,* 1992, pp. 34-38.

8. Ogilvie-Harris, D., Botsford, D., and Hawker, R. Elderly patients with hip fractures: improved outcome with the use of CareMaps with high-quality medical and nursing protocols. *Journal of Orthopaedic Trauma* 7(5):428-37, 1993.

9. Trubo, R. If this is cookbook medicine, you may like it. *Medical Economics* 70(5):69-82, Mar. 1993.

10. Southwick, K. Labs step in to help map care. *College of American Pathologists Today* 8(2):11-15, Feb. 1994.

11. Rohrer, K., Poppe, M., and Noel, L. On the scene: managed care at The Johns Hopkins Hospital. *Nursing Administration Quarterly* 7(3):54-79, 1993.

12. Migchelbrink, D., Anderson, D., Schultz, P., and Charles, C. Population-based managed care: one hospital's experience. *Nursing Administration Quarterly* 17(3):39-44, 1993.

13. Ely, B., Walker, R., and Berger, T. Case management in a small rural hospital. *Nursing Administration Quarterly* 17(3):45-53, 1993.

14. Burack, E. *The Manager's Guide to Change.* Belmont, CA: Lifetime Learning Publications, 1979.

15. Belasco, J. *Teaching the Elephant to Dance: The Manager's Guide to Empowering Change.* New York City: Penguin Books, 1991.

16. Koerner, J., Bunkers, S., and Nelson, J. Change: a professional challenge. *Nursing Administration Quarterly* 16(1):15-21, Fall 1991.

17. McKenzie, L. Critical thinking in health care supervision. *Health Care Supervision* 10(4):1-11, June 1992.

18. Harbison, J. Clinical decision making in nursing. *Journal of Advanced Nursing* 16(4):404-7, Apr. 1991.

19. Boostrom, R. *Developing Creative and Critical Thinking.* Lincolnwood, IL: National Textbook Company, 1992.

20. DeBono, E. *Six Thinking Hats.* Boston: Little, Brown, 1985.

21. Fisher, R., and Ury, W. *Getting to Yes.* New York City: Penguin Books, 1991.

22. Bueno, M., and Hwang, R. Understanding variance in hospital stay. *Nursing Management* 24(11):51–57, Nov. 1993.

23. Campbell, A., and Lakier, N. Process intervention: applying TQM to clinical care. *Healthcare Forum Journal* 35(4):81–83, July–Aug. 1992.

24. Cline, K. Clinical Pathways seen as opportunity to integrate traditional QA with CQI. *QI/TQM* 2(4):49–52, Apr. 1992.

25. Wood, R., Bailey, N., and Tilkemeier, D. Managed care: the missing link in quality improvement. *Journal of Nursing Care Quality* 6(4):55–65, July 1992.

26. Zander, K. CareMaps: the core of cost/quality care. *The New Definition* 6(3):1–3, Fall 1991.

27. Zander, K. CareMaps: quantifying, managing, and improving quality: the collaborative management of quality care. *The New Definition* 7(3):1–2, Summer 1992.

28. Zander, K. CareMaps: quantifying, managing and improving quality: using variance concurrently. *The New Definition* 7(4):1–4, Fall 1992.

29. Zander, K. CareMaps: quantifying, managing, and improving quality: the retrospective use of variance. *The New Definition* 8(1):1–3, Winter 1993.

30. Koutzes, J., and Posner, B. *Credibility.* San Francisco: Jossey-Bass Publishers, 1993, p. 25.

31. Koutzes, J., and Posner, B. *Credibility.* San Francisco: Jossey-Bass Publishers, 1993, p. 3.

32. Nolin, C., and Lang, C. *An Analysis of the Use and Effect of CareMap Tools in Medical Malpractice Litigation.* South Natick, MA: The Center for Case Management, 1994.

CareMap Development and Implementation

Kathleen M. Andolina

The creation of a CareMap tool for an identified patient population (case type) is a collaborative process involving consensus building, negotiation, and review of empirical data. In that the process is one of building a "road map" for care, it is a cartographic activity in which both science and art are recognizable elements.

CareMap tools take the clinical knowledge systematically acquired through practice and formally track it against actual care for a defined case type. However, having a technology for integrating caregiver knowledge with the practice environment does not in itself make CareMap cartography scientific. Scientific methodology must be present. When caregivers discuss interventions that correlate with outcomes, it is not unlike the scientific reasoning process used to generate hypotheses. In CareMap cartography, these "hypotheses" are tested in the actual clinical environment and through variance analysis processes that enable caregivers to make decisions about the importance of problems and the actions required for follow-through. Thus, the CareMap tool functions as the design plan for action research.

However, CareMap cartography also is an artistic endeavor in that the tool's development and implementation represents the conscious, creative effort of team members who, it could be said, write the "music" of health care. Often innovation, skill, and imagination are utilized to enhance the achievement of outcomes.

This chapter discusses the CareMap cartography process, focusing on the elements involved in forming collaborative care teams to develop and implement CareMap tools. It also addresses standards for measuring the tools' progress.

CareMap Tool Development

CareMap tool development involves the efforts of selected caregivers with recognized expertise to define the minimum action protocol that states the interventions and outcomes for a given case type.[1] Following are descriptions of the different elements involved in that process.

Setting the Stage

Before a multidisciplinary group session is convened, several important issues need to be decided. For example:

1. *The case type population requires definition.* Often the diagnosis-related group (DRG) code, procedure, or condition serves as the first step in defining the case type. It is important that the executive steering committee approve the selected population and outline a preliminary method for addressing problems as discovered in the actual management of the case type. Figure 5-1 describes examples of case type populations organized in a number of descriptive forms.
2. *The length of stay (LOS) parameters should be provided.* Length of stay serves as a basic financial indicator and also assists caregivers in determining appropriate outcomes for the allotted time frame.
3. *The roles for developing and managing the CareMap tool from initiation through implementation must be established.* (See figure 5-2.)
4. *Composition of the collaborative/author team and the care areas they will represent requires thoughtful coordination.* The invitation and scheduling of caregivers, administrators, and department heads most identified with care for the defined case type, including at least one physician, are important first steps. Team size is of minimal concern at this time, recognizing that it is better to be inclusive rather than exclusive. However, caregiver mix is important. The degree and quality of caregiver interactions with the case type population in practice are influential to the final product. Problematic issues such as low team morale, cynicism, or poor communication will become magnified within mapping sessions. Thus, preliminary team building is a better investment in these situations, saving the mapping session for synthesis of the map content. In addition, the physician participation is essential at initial development sessions.[2] If the physician cannot attend the session, it is best for the facilitator to reschedule it.

Facilitating the Development Session

Facilitating the development session requires both leadership flexibility and structure. There is no one way to produce a map. Each CareMap tool will reflect the author group, the facilitator style, and the setting in which the case type population is treated. However, there are some general guidelines for accomplishing productive sessions and making the most of valuable caregiver time.

Figure 5-1. Descriptive Categories for Case Type Populations

Descriptive Category	Examples
DRG	209 Total Knee Replacement 430 Depression, Psychosis
Procedures	Surgical Hip TURP Coronary Artery Bypass Graft (CABG) Cardiac Catheterization
Conditions	Congestive Heart Failure (CHF) Chronic Obstructive Pulmonary Disease (COPD) Diabetes Asthma
Phase or Segment of Care	Neonatal 39–41 Weeks Adolescent Inpatient (psychiatric) Emergency Department, Acute Myocardial Infarct

Figure 5-2. Roles, Tasks, and Responsibilities That Support a Productive Mapping Process

Roles for Developing and Managing CareMap Tools	Definition of Tasks and Responsibilities
Project Manager	Provides the general structure for the CareMap Project, articulates with the executive steering committee, often facilitates CareMap development sessions
Facilitator	Project manager or clinical leader who facilitates a development session, forms goals for the session, guides the group to meet the goals of the work group and identifies issues/obstacles in completing the map.
Author Group	Participants who are connected to the population of concern as either clinical, service, or support providers. In addition, a rotating membership might be formed to address occasional information needs such as executives/administrators, utilization managers, educators, consultants, and so forth.
Team Manager	Team manager is a designated person who addresses the functional needs of the author group. These needs include scheduling, memos, managing the draft in production of the map and distribution to authors, and so forth.
Physician Participant	Physician who participates in the map development session. Shares perspective on focus of care, discharge criteria, recommendations for resource utilization and patterns of care. At more involved levels, the physician participates as author and liaison to physician peers, writes companion order sets to go with the map, collaboratively reviews aggregate data, writes policies about routine interactions in patient care assessment using the map, and conducts research.
Patient and Family Focus Groups	Using a focus group approach, former patients and families can comment on the language and content, reviewing it for understandability, patient-centeredness, participation and continuity, and so forth.

Selecting the Facilitator

The facilitator keeps the group process moving. Caregivers or leaders who have expertise in work group facilitation, issue prioritization, pace setting, and time management are valuable in the role. Although the facilitator is often the project manager, the role could as effectively be filled by a clinical leader from within the author group. This person adds credibility as a clinical expert. He or she also provides increased availability to the group and is an expert resource for the team when the project manager is not available.

The ability to generate spirited discussion and encourage curiosity without straying from the purpose of creating a map is helpful in establishing a successful collaborative framework. It enables caregivers to feel free to question each other about their rationale for proposing actions and to work as a team to engage in problem solving. Supporting this creative, inquisitive environment reinforces positive patterns of multidisciplinary communication and makes for an extraordinary work experience.

Setting the Agenda

Getting bogged down with details can be distracting to the group process. Over time, the team and the facilitator will learn when perseveration is helpful or when it is not, and will utilize lengthy discussion accordingly. Thus, setting an agenda for both initial development and revision sessions will be helpful. (See figure 5-3.) An agenda serves to keep session members on target in terms of both the topic to be discussed and the discussion time to be allotted to each topic. At the end of each session, time should be provided to focus member attention on the next steps and to propose agenda items for future meetings. This allows the facilitator to encourage team participation in designing and managing care for the defined case type. It is important for author teams to understand the first development session is not the last. In fact, initially, it may require four to six hours of meetings to establish a map with content that the team expresses confidence in and finally feels ready to pilot on a test number of case patients.

Determining the Time Frame

There is a well-known commandment in health care that can be stated something like this: Thou shalt not waste my time. Yet this rule is broken every day through overscheduling, underpreparation, and lack of team focus on productive ends. A mapping session is best structured with an agenda and limited to an hour and a half. If sessions run too long, caregivers become tired, bored, or anxious about getting back to their work. It is important to respect time parameters by starting and stopping on time. By observing this unspoken rule, meetings will be kept focused and stimulating.

Figure 5-3. Sample Agenda for CareMap Development Session

Initial CareMap Development Session (2 hours maximum)

1. Orientation (5–10 minutes)
   a. Introduce members and explain the process.

2. Profiling the case type (25–35 minutes)
   a. Discuss reasons for choosing this patient population, including a review of case type data, level of interest, and other key factors.
   b. Discuss symptoms for admission, anatomy and physiology, discharge criteria (provided by physician leader).
   c. Define other problems or focus: physiologic, psychosocial, knowledge, functional, and complications or obstacles (other disciplines).
   d. Discuss issues such as present LOS (fiscal/UR), exclusions from map, caregivers/areas involved, reasons for the map.

3. Completing the process (35 minutes)
   a. Set up the grid (see figure 5-5): time and location sequence (*y* axis) and care elements (*x* axis).
   b. Complete columns 1 and 2, discussing interventions and outcomes.
   c. Fill in across rows where possible.
   d. Identify issues, potential variances, and obstacles.

4. Next steps (15 minutes)
   a. Ask team to focus on these patients between now and the next meeting; refer to literature, standards for more detailed content.
   b. Consider elements such as who will use the map and what suggestions can be thought of to pilot the tool.
   c. Set date, time, and agenda for next meeting.

Subsequent CareMap Development Session (2 hours)

1. Discuss changes to be made on the critical path section, new ideas, and so on.
2. Link discharge criteria to physician list of symptoms/issues/nursing diagnosis. Begin setting intermediate goals, first at critical points, then in-between.
3. Do a cross-check to ensure that intermediate goals match the interventions and vice versa.
4. Pilot the tool off-the-record with 5 to 10 patients, then meet again to review results and revise.

Setting up the Meeting Room

The most effective setup for seating session members is around a circular table. This creates a face-to-face setting in which caregivers can become familiar with each other as equal contributors to the process. If a round table is unavailable or not large enough to seat everyone comfortably, an option is to angle rows of chairs facing the facilitator. It is important to avoid amphitheaterlike arrangements, podiums, and microphones.

Little equipment is required. Markers, large sheets of paper, tape, and a white board or chalkboard should be all that are necessary to conduct session business. Any drafts produced probably will be messy and confusing, so it is best to ask a volunteer to keep discussion notes that can later be typewritten.

Conducting the Initial CareMap Development Session

A successful initial CareMap development session will focus team members on the work they have been assembled to do. After a brief orientation, time should be devoted to profiling the case type for which the CareMap is being written, identifying and prioritizing problems, anticipating potential variances, and so on.

Orienting Session Members

It would be extremely helpful to take a few minutes at the beginning of the session to orient team members to the purpose of the meeting. Normally, orientation would consist of making introductions, outlining expectations, and reviewing the meeting structure. This phase of the meeting will go a long way toward ensuring that all members understand the process and know what is expected of them.

Profiling the Case Type

A starting point for authoring a CareMap for a defined case type would be to work up a profile of that patient population. This is useful for orienting team members who are less familiar with the case type as well as ensuring that everyone is starting from the same knowledge base. The team's physician leader will play a major role in this endeavor. Using his or her teaching and leadership qualities, the physician can share his or her knowledge in terms of understanding, approaching, and evaluating patients in this case type. Some physicians may elect to support and review their discussion with audiovisuals or handouts. In any event, sufficient time should be allowed for full discussion of the patient population that is the object of the CareMap. The payback of this investment for team members is twofold: First, it clarifies the map's purpose and language and, second, it improves caregiver understanding of the care approach used by the physician leader for this case type.

Thus, discussion of the population profile and the clinician's experience, as well as diagnostic indicators and clinical algorithms, will serve to clarify the characteristics that define the case type in question. Other information that communicates the description of this patient population includes the prescribed LOS, geographic care areas, and criteria for screening and detecting patients appropriate for the map. In addition, it is important to outline what comorbidities or complications are beyond the scope of the CareMap. For example, cognitive impairment may occur in association with pneumonia, but not often enough to include it in the map for pneumonia. It is thus excluded from the pneumonia map. Any exclusions often become different maps altogether or future derivative maps. Following are illustrations of the criteria for case type inclusion and exclusion for an AIDS CareMap tool:

- *Inclusion criteria:* Adult AIDS patients with T cells < 200, presenting with opportunistic infections, anorexia/wasting syndrome, significant other/caretaker

absence, recent loss of job, with possible dementia, suicidal or assaultive idea-
tion. Reason for admission was deemed to be palliative but restorative.
- *Exclusion criteria:* AIDS patients who are vent dependent or arrive in the emergency room with acute trauma (motor vehicle accident or gunshot, for example)

At some point during the initial discussion, it will be important to ask team members *what it is they want the CareMap tool to do.* This helps them to clarify reasons
and rationale for using the map and determines how the map results will be evaluated. Goals for a single map are more specific and operational than global CareMap
initiative goals. Figure 5-4 illustrates the relationship between map and system goals
as well as the short- and long-term goals for the individual map.

Defining Intermediate Outcomes

Generally, caregivers have little difficulty defining problems, interventions, and discharge outcomes; however, defining intermediate outcomes is more difficult and time-
consuming. Therefore, proceeding in a way that builds on the success of the discussion of easier components provides positive momentum for addressing more complex
variables of care.

Figure 5-5 shows a grid that team members might use to focus on these care variables. Starting at the top of the grid under "Problems/Focus," team members list the
problems associated with the case type and, if possible, prioritize them. Next, they
state the discharge criteria (which at this stage do not have to be directly connected
to the problem/focus areas). Then, they describe interventions within the time frames
and critical path care categories. Tasks and interventions are placed within the category
that best matches their action. For example, vital signs, pulse oximetry, or central
venous pressures (CVPs) are tasks that best fit in the "Assessments" category, whereas
complete blood counts (CBCs), pulmonary function tests (PFTs), and chest X rays better fit the "Tests" category. Time and location intervals on the map can be defined
by day, geographical area, or criteria-based phase of care (that is, phase 1/evaluation,
phase 2/stabilization, and so forth). Finally, team members add the intermediate outcome statements. It is important to keep the outcomes stated in patient-centered language, rather than in caregiver goal terms.

Reviewing the Care Areas Involved

A review of the journey that patients and families take through the maze of health
care services, departments, and areas serves as the basis for defining the interval
columns within the map. Figure 5-6 uses interval columns to show: (a) how multiple
locations can be organized within a single time span, (b) how care areas can have their
own column within a single time frame, (c) phases of care within a single time frame,
and (d) phases of care spanning multiple visits. Although the columns define the care
areas and time sequences more precisely, accountability for tasks and outcomes within
the intervals should be equally precise. (See figure 5-7.)

Identifying Problems

The terminology used on the CareMap to describe problems (or other focus area) is
a pivotal point for team discussion. For instance, if nursing diagnosis is to be the framework for identifying problems within nursing, how well the team understands the meaning, scope, and comprehensiveness of nursing diagnosis is key to the terminology's
acceptance and utility. Alternate or derivative language may be the solution. For example, on a CareMap written by a team in one hospital, patients and families who had
difficulty with end-stage cancer care decisions about extraordinary medical measures

Figure 5-4. Differentiating Author Team Goals from the Larger CareMap Program Initiative Goals

CareMap System Goals	CareMap Author Team Goals
1. Involve all clinical care settings with high-volume, high-cost case types in the CareMap initiative where possible. 2. Provide cost-effective, coordinated care of high quality to the populations served by the facility. 3. Demonstrate improved patient satisfaction.	**Posttraumatic Stress Disorder (PTSD) Author Team** **Short-term:** 1. Define and coordinate knowledge regarding PTSD care and treatment. 2. Decrease LOS (from 10 to 9 days). 3. State outcomes. **Long-term:** 1. Integrate the inpatient map with the day treatment map for PTSD. 2. Develop map for patient/family education.
	Femoral Popliteal Bypass Graft (FPBG) Author Team **Short-term:** 1. Reduce unnecessary variation in practice. 2. Increase interdisciplinary communication and collaboration. 3. Test how well the map guides order writing. **Long-term:** 1. Patient/family map. 2. Integrate standing orders into the map.
	Pyelonephritis Author Team **Short-term:** 1. Define and measure discharge outcomes. 2. Increase interdisciplinary communication and collaboration. 3. Reduce unnecessary variation in practice, compare uses of tests and antibiotics to a control team of pyelo patients, and evaluate differences and outcomes.

Figure 5-5. The CareMap Grid and Elements to Complete in a Development Session

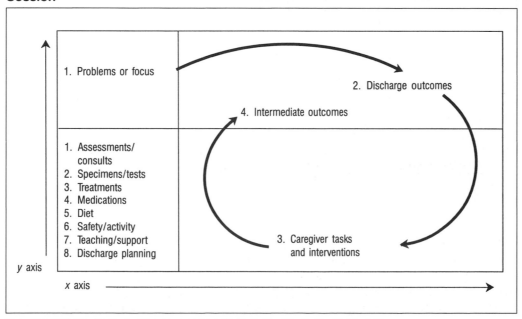

121

Figure 5-6. CareMap Columns Used to Display Time Progression and Location Changes

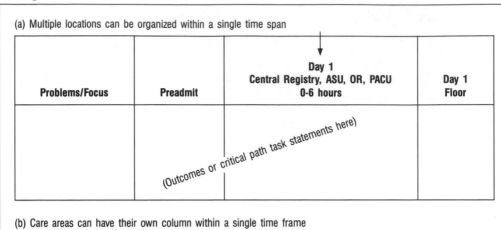

(a) Multiple locations can be organized within a single time span

Problems/Focus	Preadmit	Day 1 Central Registry, ASU, OR, PACU 0-6 hours	Day 1 Floor
		(Outcomes or critical path task statements here)	

(b) Care areas can have their own column within a single time frame

Problems/Focus	Day 1 Emergency Department 0-2 hours	Day 1 Operating Room	Day 1 PACU	Day 1 Unit
		(Outcomes or critical path task statements here)		

(c) Phases of care within a single time frame

	Emergency Department 0-4 hours		
Physicians Office	Triage	Diagnostics	Assessment and Diagnosis
		(Outcomes or critical path task statements here)	

(d) Phases of care spanning multiple visits

	Phase I: Assessment/Orientation		
Telephone Contact	Visit 1	Visit 2	Visit 3
		(Outcomes or critical path task statements here)	

Figure 5-7.   Defining Accountability for Tasks and Outcomes within the Grid Cells

1. Care Element ↓	Day 3 (Post-Op Day 2)
	Interventions
Nutrition/Diet	Dietary: Determine caloric needs
Activity	RN/PT: Increase CPM as patient tolerates PT: Transfer patient to chair with walker or crutches RN: Continue mobilizing patient bed to chair
Discharge Planning	Discharge planning RN: Collaborates with physician to plan post-op care

were captured under the heading "Altered Family Process." After some experience with the map, it was discovered that there was caregiver confusion about the exact meaning of that term. Thus, the problem statement was changed to "Family Decisional Conflict: End-Stage Care." Equally important is how well the patient/family understands the terminology on the map and how the map is to be used. For example, if clinicians use technical jargon to describe care on the CareMap tool, patients and families who are given the map will have difficulty understanding how the map applies to them directly and may also become concerned if they are at variance with the goals as stated on the map. Often patient versions of the CareMap tool are provided for teaching purposes.

Anticipating Potential Variances

Listing subcategories on a piece of paper under the heading of "Variance" is helpful in assisting team members to predetermine their own obstacles within the case type. The categories of "patient/family," "caregiver," "system," and "community" not only help caregivers discriminate between the reasons for variance but also can lead to problem solving before a problem occurs. For example, in the case type for AIDS, the team predicted that there would be variance in meeting self-care outcomes in cases where the patient had AIDS-related dementia. Team members discovered that they had questions about the recognition, etiology, and treatment of dementia in this population. Instead of listing dementia as a problem or focus area on the Care-Map, they opted to screen for it as a patient variance, propose a process for addressing it as an add-on problem, and trend the results. Meanwhile, a neurologist and a psychiatrist would be called on to respond to team member questions, a literature review would be requested on AIDS-related dementia, and a DRG coding report would be undertaken to provide information about incidences of dementia in admitted AIDS patients.

In another situation, a CareMap team attempted to address a common "caregiver" variance. The cerebral vascular accident (CVA) team began to address how a critical point in care occurred at three to four days poststroke. At this time, although the information about prognosis was becoming clearer, caregivers were fragmented, communicating poorly, and the families were complaining that they were getting conflicting reports on the patient's status. This resulted in family dissatisfaction and uninformed decision making about care decisions related to the patient. The team established the outcome standard that members would meet three to four days poststroke to address specific questions about clinical, functional, and family issues. The standard was incorporated into the CareMap and the team set a date to begin the intervention, expecting to reconvene after five patients to discuss the outcome effect.

Addressing Larger Care Issues

It would be rare if persistent system problems did not come up during the discussion in cartography sessions. Generally, these problems pose serious barriers to achieving cost and quality outcomes and expend team energy and effort. Discussing these issues is an important function in that it involves caregivers and administration coming together to solve organizationwide problems. CareMap programs now offer a structure for detecting and managing these issues in a comprehensive way.

All larger care issues that come up during discussion should be recorded on a sheet of paper under the heading "Issues." Sometimes an issue can be resolved immediately if the appropriate person is in the room at the time the issue is detected. For example, in one situation a physician agreed to use consistent wording in his diet orders after hearing a dietitian clarify the wording for diet orders for cardiac patients. Other times, issues that arise during discussion may be managed differently. For example, when COPD team members at one institution discussed the difficulty they experienced with patients who were in progressive decline, they explored the possibility of an ethics review to help identify levels of care and medical intervention with this case type. They elected to keep the issue on the "active" list and address it at the next team meeting. In other instances, a system issue may be identified but not solvable at the team level. For example, a Veterans Administration CareMap team felt patients could be more quickly admitted from the emergency department. Because of the long-standing tradition of admitting patients based on service-connected rating rather than on acuity or treatability, there were consistent delays in admissions as patients with greater service ratings were admitted first. This made it difficult to guarantee smooth, predictable transitions between care areas and led to delayed outcomes. And in yet other cases, discovering issues gave the team a cause. For example, in one hospital the use of outdated criteria for preoperative testing standards by the peer review organization (PRO) resulted in continued expensive and unnecessary patient testing, despite the lack of clinical necessity. Further, if the charts did not meet PRO standards, there was the distinct possibility of chart denial and lost revenue for the hospital. Thus, the team developing a CareMap for cataract surgery concluded that a formal strategy beyond hospital-based interventions was needed to advocate for change.

Closing the Session

Before the session is closed, team members should be asked to discuss what they see as the next step. The facilitator models self-management by explaining what next steps will be taken in terms of map production. For example, he or she may inform the team that a typewritten draft will be provided for review and editing. Another way to close the session is to ask team members what they would like to have happen at the next session and if they feel that additional individuals should be invited. Establishing a tentative or fixed date for the next meeting and proposing an agenda will help keep the team's momentum going.

Implementation of the CareMap Tool

Once the initial draft of the CareMap tool has been produced, it is ready to be implemented. The first stage of implementation is to pilot the map.

The Pilot Process

The pilot process is the method for testing the CareMap tool. This process requires management at the program management level, rather than at the author team level.

The larger structure is required to address issues that will pertain to multiple CareMaps and author teams. This structure allows decision making to occur consistently and efficiently as maps are implemented facilitywide. The pilot process is complex and requires that a number of decisions be made. The who, what, when, where, and why of the pilot process require definition. The details are often subject to considerable debate and indecision. Figure 5-8 lists some common start-up questions and succinct answers that give better definition to a project as it proceeds.

Clarifying the goals of the pilot will help shape its expectations. For example, which of the following goals will the pilot test:

- The content of the map for appropriateness to case type and involve only a few selected staff
- The content of the map for appropriateness to case type and involve all staff

Figure 5-8. Common Start-Up Questions and Short Answers for a CareMap Tool Pilot

Common Start-Up Questions	The Short Answer
1. Where is the CareMap stored?	Eventually in the medical record.
2. What do I do when a patient is admitted? Who places the patient on the CareMap?	Collaborate with the MD and place the map into the chart.
3. What happens if the CareMap does not fit the patient?	Customize the map to the patient or take the patient off the map if there are too many complications. Revert to previous documentation system.
4. How many patients are placed on the CareMap during the trial?	Usually no more than 5 to 10 and for no longer than 2 to 6 weeks.
5. What do I do with the form when the patient is discharged or transferred?	Send it to the team manager or project manager for review and collection of data.
6. Who is responsible for reading the CareMap, when, and how often?	Review of the CareMap can be done at MD rounds, admission, critical points of variance, and (at a minimum) change of shift.
7. When can I expect to learn the results of the CareMap trial?	As soon as the team reconvenes and reviews actual maps and summarized data.
8. When do we start using the CareMap for real?	After there is sufficient confidence in its utility and accuracy.
9. What if I have an idea for a CareMap?	Survey interest from multidisciplinary colleagues and coordinate development with the project manager.
10. Are we going to use case managers?	Maybe, depends on how well the map coordinates caregivers and assists in addressing variances.
11. What happens to the other documentation system, and how does it interact with CareMap tools?	Maps can cover between 50 and 80 percent of populations of patients. Where there is no map for a patient diagnosis, there needs to be an alternative documentation system.
12. Can I do anything wrong during the pilot?	Yes, ignore it.
13. What do the collaborative care teams say are the goals for their maps?	These are defined by the teams in terms of short- and long-term goals. These should be open to other teams to view.
14. How long does the pilot last?	Until either five patients have been placed on maps or two to four weeks pass, whichever comes first.

- Both content of the map for appropriateness and utility as a system of documentation, as well as familiarize all caregivers with the tool
- The content of the map for appropriateness to case type, utility as a system of documentation, and staff role in variance data collection

Once the basic goals are established, other strategies will be required to address certain questions including:

- Will the CareMap tool be tested in all the care areas or on one unit or floor?
- Which physicians will use the map?
- Will those physicians include members from an internal group practice, house officers, residents, or private admitting physicians?
- Will a variance tool be tested at this time?
- Will variance reasons be predefined or will variance be collected on every outcome or intervention statement?
- Who will collect variance data, and who will analyze them?
- How will the information be routed, and what actions on variances will be expected during the pilot phase?

The answers to these questions will determine the scope of the strategy used to prepare caregivers and to measure the pilot's results. In some instances, the executive steering committee, pilot task force, or CareMap author teams themselves will address the pilot implementation questions.

It is prudent to consider a route for multidisciplinary acceptance of the CareMap tool. Figure 5-9 is a flowchart showing the "ratification" process used at St. Francis Hospital in Poughkeepsie, New York, to involve physicians and department directors in signing off on CareMap tools.

Increased Independence from the Facilitator

For CareMap development teams to manage the quality of care for the case type, they must strive to be self-governing. Every instance of team authority and leadership in

Figure 5-9.   Process for Authoring, Ratifying, and Revising CareMap Tools

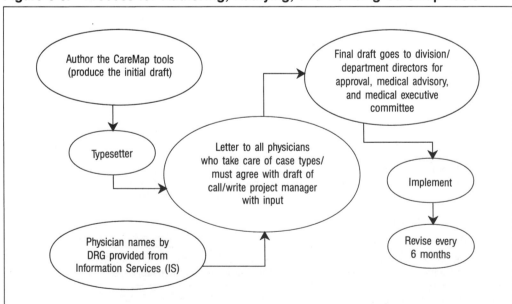

Reprinted, with permission, from L. LaRotunda, St. Francis Hospital, Poughkeepsie, New York.

determining CareMap content, facilitating the process, and evaluating the outcome brings the team closer to realizing the promise of collaborative, outcome-based practice. Seeking and grooming cofacilitators, or team members skilled in team leadership, is advisable as early in the process as possible. In some instances it is helpful to appoint a "team manager," a consistent or rotating person who can schedule initial/revision meetings, define the team reports or minutes to be prepared, and generally support the team as it develops momentum toward goal achievement and self-management.

Dissemination of Knowledge

If the CareMap tool is to have long-range impact and increase the likelihood of making change stick, it must be shared. Increasingly, caregivers are willing to share outcomes discovered in the practice of clinical art and science, via CareMap tools. Outcome information and successes may be shared and disseminated through publications, internal and external marketing, program evaluations, or seminar-style presentations. Those clinicians actually using maps in daily practice make credible and knowledgeable speakers on topics related to outcomes practice. The best time to begin communicating results occurs after some experience with development and use of the maps through several revisions. This can be up to a year or two into an initiative.

Evaluation of CareMap Cartography

As mentioned earlier, CareMap cartography is both an art and a science. Its evaluation process may be looked at in the same way. CareMap results are most easily evaluated when there is an external set of established criteria; however, in the instance of art these criteria are often shifting and culturally determined. The judges of the artistic nature of the cartography experience reside only in the CareMap author team. For one team artistic accomplishment may be evident in the tool design, whereas for another it may lie in the ability to creatively manage variance.

On the other hand, the CareMap tool with its content and variance system represents a scientific method for predicting the results of clinical practice. Though static in form, it is not static in process. This presents difficulty in managing a central issue in research methodology—that of establishing control. Related to this are other troublesome questions about the results of a clinical methodology as applied to a case type. For example:

- How precisely defined is the case type?
- How representative are the aggregate data to other similar case types?
- Is the methodology reproducible, and can the results be generalized?
- Are the concepts and terms used within the map operationally defined?
- Do the stated interventions support causative or correlational predictions made in the outcome statements?
- How representative is the content on the CareMap of the team effort versus a reflection of a single, more vocal author?

Where possible, it is preferable that the CareMap team build in control for the purpose of learning about the initiative's true effectiveness. Thus, regular (at least quarterly) review of the map is recommended to maintain the integrity and relevancy of its content, respond to practice changes or new knowledge, and review the status of quality and cost outcomes.

Following are descriptions of other stakeholders in the evaluation of CareMap cartography. These include the Joint Commission on Accreditation of Healthcare Organizations (JCAHO), patients and families, the health care facility itself, and managed care companies.

The JCAHO Survey Process

Perhaps the most practical standard for measuring the promise of CareMap accomplishment is through the JCAHO survey process, where health care organizations invite a national team to review operations and systems compared to JCAHO quality criteria. The JCAHO's focus in its Agenda for Change[3] centers on devising standards that measure organizational support and commitment for effective, efficient, and well-performed care. (See figure 5-10.)

The JCAHO recognizes that "patient outcomes will be improved only by increasing the effectiveness and efficiency of organizational functions."[4] Because of its basis in the real work of health care professionals and its focus on outcomes, the CareMap tool qualifies as a method for assisting organizations in actualizing the goals of their mission. If a mission statement could be inferred from the JCAHO standards, it would read as follows:

> It is the mission of this organization to provide effective, efficient, and appropriate care that is available, timely, continuous, safe, respectful, and caring for 100 percent of the patients and families we serve.

CareMap tools and systems provide the structure for efficient, timely, continuous, and appropriate care. The "safe, respectful, and caring" aspects depend less on the tool than on the individuals within the organization who will use it. Paper tools and team structures can not, and should not, replace the impact made by individuals within a system.

Figure 5-10. JCAHO Emphasis in the Agenda for Change Initiative and Correlating Features in CareMap Tools and Systems

Agenda for Change Emphasis	CareMap Tools and Systems
Outcomes over methods	Outcomes stated across time, care area Outcomes listed as intermediate and discharge statements
Recognition for facility uniqueness.	Maps and systems are customized to facility resources, culture, and mission.
Improvement is continuous.	Maps/systems are not static, but dynamic tools that change when practice changes and utilize variance data to guide and monitor improvement initiatives.
Functionally grouped standards: • Assessment of patients • Treatment of patients • Operative/invasive procedures • Education of patients and families • Leadership • Management of information • Improving organizational performance	CareMaps/Systems: • Predict assessment activities for populations of patients. • Treatments are defined, timed, and accountabilities clarified. • Critical quality interventions can be organized on maps for procedures, particularly in the preparation of patients and systems for the procedure. • Patient/family versions of maps better prepare patients for the care experience. • Maps are tools for implementing leadership mission and vision for patient care services. • Maps often streamline documentation and provide the data base for CQI and UM initiatives. • Variance analysis is the method for trending and action planning based on measured data.
Statistical process control techniques familiar to all members of a team.	All team members learn the language of outcomes measurement using maps and variance, are able to communicate with other teams, and use the same language to address system improvements.

Patients and Families

Other stakeholders in the evaluation process are patients and their families. Patient and family evaluation of maps is indistinguishable from their evaluation of actual care. Was the care experience minimally disruptive? Was it perceived as seamless? Was the map a useful communication tool, and did patients and their families feel prepared for the care events? Did the actual outcomes match the map and, if not, was the explanation to the patient reasonable and acceptable? This kind of evaluation can be useful at discharge or in the form of a follow-up survey. In addition, small focus groups of former patients can be used to review and comment on the map. This involves the patient and family on a retrospective level to provide a valuable feedback mechanism for revising language and content.

Health Care Organizations

Organizations that authorize map initiatives will be interested to see how well the maps achieved expected results in several areas. Were the overall program goals achieved within the organizational time frame predicted? Are annual and regular map review mechanisms in place that not only address the original rationale for the program but also track individual map progress? Were systems issues effectively managed using the data detected from a map? Positive indicators in these realms indicate successful use of the map and effective systems for managing variance. In addition, maps also can be evaluated on the basis of their value as benchmarks for comparison with other similar-resourced hospitals.

Managed Care Companies

Managed care companies (third-party payers, HMOs, group purchasers, and so forth) often negotiate contracts with health care organizations based on the following provisos: costs of care, emphasis on prevention and wellness, numbers of primary care providers, and quality of care. In addition, managed care companies are beginning to ask whether health care organizations are using maps and critical paths to guide care. How well maps begin to address and manage care along lines of cost, quality, wellness, and prevention will determine their future utility in managed care systems.

Conclusion

CareMap cartography is the process of creating a road map to better manage the costs, quality, and outcomes of patient care. In effect, it is both an artistic and scientific endeavor—artistic because it represents a conscious, creative effort on the part of the CareMap author team and scientific because it involves tracking clinically acquired data against actual care to measure its effectiveness.

The first stage in producing a CareMap tool is to bring together a team of caregivers who can combine their expertise to map a care plan for a defined patient population. Once the session is physically arranged, a facilitator must be assigned, caregivers oriented, and a case type profile developed. This puts team members on an equal footing and serves to identify any problems with the plan and anticipate any variances in care. Once a CareMap has been written, the next stage is to implement it through creation of a pilot program that the team can monitor and evaluate without outside help.

CareMap cartography evaluation also is an artistic and scientific endeavor, depending on team creativity and the controls built in by the team to measure the intiative's effectiveness. However, evaluation goes beyond the controls set by the team. JCAHO standards, patients and families, the organization itself, and managed care companies all offer measurement criteria.

Although thus far CareMap cartography may not be a rigorous process, its results appear to be compelling. These include better teamwork, consistent care evaluation, patient-centeredness, and a focus on effective and efficient care.

References

1. Zander, K. *The New Definition* 6(3), 1991.

2. Zander, K. Physicians, CareMaps, and collaboration. *The New Definition* 7(1):1–3, Winter 1992.

3. Joint Commission on Accreditation of Healthcare Organizations. *1994 Accreditation Manual for Hospitals.* Vol. 1. Oakbrook Terrace, IL: JCAHO, 1993.

4. JCAHO.

CHAPTER SIX

The Uses of Variance

Patricia Potter

Clearly the purchasers of health care are pursuing quality and value for their money — the provision of necessary care at reasonable cost. Nash[1] warns that if health care cannot be measured or differentiated on the basis of quality, businesses will be forced to conclude that all medical care is of equal quality and will buy it on the basis of price alone. In the past, quality has been an enigma, defined on the basis of criteria that fail to reflect the outcomes of effective patient–clinician interaction. In other words, traditional criteria such as fall rates, morbidity and mortality, and infection rates do not provide the detail necessary to reveal the link between clinical interventions and good care outcomes.

An outcome is the result of a process, and a *good* outcome is a result that achieves the goal of the process.[2] When a hospital identifies the means to reach care outcomes in a formalized way, it has successfully defined the quality of its product. If the care outcomes are successfully achieved, a hospital that simultaneously reduces costs and garners patient satisfaction will become a leader in the industry.

This chapter discusses the clinical uses of variance and the retrospective uses of variance for quality improvement. It also discusses the various legal ramifications of variance collection and reporting.

The Concept of Variance

Variance is a crucial aspect of critical path/CareMap implementation and success. The following subsections describe critical paths/CareMaps, provide a definition of variance, and suggest an approach to variance analysis.

Critical Paths/CareMaps

Patient care is a complex phenomenon involving the contributions of caregivers from a variety of health care disciplines. Critical paths/CareMaps represent the collaboration of clinical experts who have defined the minimum clinical standards or essential components of care for every patient with a given diagnosis.[3] Each CareMap defines the problems that patients in a defined case type typically encounter and thus directs the development of a comprehensive approach to their care. When caregivers collaborate, a picture evolves describing what interventions are to be delivered and what results or outcomes can be anticipated over the course of a predicted length of stay (LOS).

Additionally, critical paths/CareMaps describe the clinical work of health care professionals as it relates to patients' and families' measurable outcomes of care.[4] Well-developed CareMaps identify the patient problems and associated clinical interventions needed to avoid adverse effects of care (for example, wound infection), improve patient physiologic outcomes (for example, range of motion), reduce pathologic signs and symptoms (for example, anxiety), and improve the patient's functional state or well-being (for example, ability to climb stairs).

In order for a health care organization to become accountable for delivering high-quality care, it must be able to provide three sets of information: evidence of continuous quality improvement (CQI), outcomes management, and clinical practice standards or guidelines.[5] When integrated into the total quality improvement process, a CareMap provides a model for outcomes management and delivery of a higher quality of care to patients.

A well-designed critical path will capture 30 to 70 percent of patients within a given population. If a bell-shaped curve is applied to a defined case type, it can be anticipated that approximately 30 to 70 percent will follow the recommended course outlined in the CareMap, whereas the remaining patients will either recover more quickly or face some sort of delay in recovery. Despite the efforts of a multidisciplinary team to identify the best process and outcomes of care for a patient population, there will always be opportunities for improvement.

Defining Variance

Variances (also called *exceptions*) are the unexpected events that occur during patient care—events that are different from what is predicted on the CareMap. *Variance analysis* gives caregivers a mechanism that can be used to study variations of care using a CareMap and to identify ways to continually improve processes and outcomes. As a result, the bell-shaped curve shifts to the right. (See figure 6-1.)

Despite the intent to define the essential components of care, there still is variation in how care will be delivered and how patients will respond. Variation is always present in processes, products, and people.[6] For example, a patient's body temperature fluctuates over a 24-hour period, or a patient's motivation to perform physical therapy routines will vary according to levels of fatigue, motivation, or pain perceived. The point-to-point differences observed over time (the variation) are caused by multiple factors.

Zander has defined variance as a deviation from the expected patient/family intermediate goals, outcomes, and staff interventions outlined on the critical path/CareMap.[7] Variance may be positive or negative. *Positive variance* occurs when patients progress toward projected outcomes earlier than anticipated, when select interventions such as pain medication administration are unnecessary, or when interventions such as patient education can successfully begin at an earlier stage. *Negative variance* occurs when either patients fail to meet projected outcomes, there is a delay in meeting outcomes, or there is a need for additional interventions previously unplanned.

Understanding variance over time is key to recognizing and using exceptions or differences observed for the purpose of continual improvement.[8] In the case of CareMaps, variance is the most important tool in understanding the effects of care and making the necessary changes to achieve the very best outcomes. Members of the clinical team who develop the CareMap review variance trends for groups of patients. They look at values falling outside the expected range that indicate some special circumstance or event. For example, variance trends may reveal the need to introduce a change in clinical therapies or to recognize the reoccurrence of a specific complication. A well-designed CareMap system allows caregivers to identify variances

Figure 6-1. Bell Curve Distribution Showing Effect of Managed Care Model Using CareMap

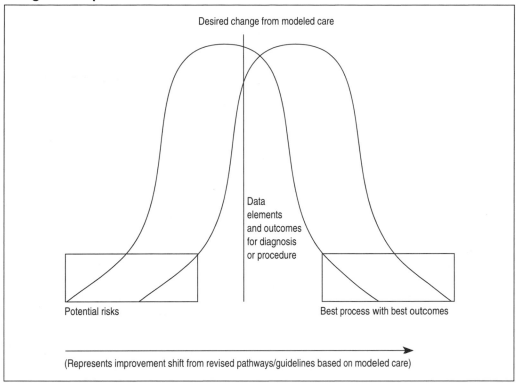

and provides the information needed to appropriately change the way care is delivered. The concept is simple: Caregivers must evaluate what works and what requires refinement or improvement to achieve higher quality at an affordable price.

Constructing an Approach to Variance Analysis

Development of a critical path/CareMap is relatively easy if the right players are involved. The clinicians responsible for the management of select patient populations know the interventions to provide, the day-to-day outcomes that measure the successful management of a patient, and the thresholds of time periods within which interventions and outcomes occur. However, over time clinicians may not be aware of their aggregate success. They may not know the recurring trends that suggest necessary changes to the approach of care. When a CareMap system is developed within an organization, a critical early step is to identify how variance will be defined, monitored, and evaluated. To analyze whether changes are truly needed in the CareMap or in the approach to care, caregivers must have accurate and meaningful data.

Typically, the executive steering committee has responsibility for determining how variance is to be incorporated into the organization's CQI program. Making that determination depends on answering certain key questions. For example:

- What type of variance information is desired? (for example, all occurrences of variance or only outcomes at variance)
- Who will record variance? (for example, nursing staff only or all care providers)
- How will variance be collected and reported? (for example, will it be integrated in the documentation system for retrieval or collected retrospectively in chart reviews)

- What will be the process for analyzing variance and making recommendations for changes in the CareMaps? (for example, will analysis be conducted by the teams of staff who develop the CareMap or by a separate quality improvement department)

Determining the type of variance data to collect is crucial. The Health Care Advisory Board[9] has reported that CareMap models often fail in organizations that become gridlocked with data. A large volume of variance data centralized for routine data collection can create a situation in which caregivers have so much information to review that they are disinclined to take corrective action. And as more and more CareMaps are introduced into the system, the volume of data can quickly become overwhelming. Thus, caregivers may find it too time-consuming to analyze information about trends in patient care, ultimately resulting in an erosion of their commitment to the CareMap system.

Zander has recommended that organizations track variances from 100 percent of intermediate goals and outcomes and 100 percent of key tasks deemed crucial to outcome achievement.[10] In other words, all outcomes incorporated into a CareMap should be tracked as well as those interventions most likely to influence a patient's progress. In the case of a chemotherapy patient, key interventions might include hydration and administration of antiemetics, while outcomes will include absence of emesis. This approach prevents a CareMap team from looking at all variances. A well-designed CareMap will include the outcomes and goals that caregivers have prioritized as essential to a patient's recovery.

However, the selection of key tasks may be more difficult. If the CareMap team trusts the tool as representing best practice, it becomes easier to identify key events or interventions. Examples of key tasks applicable to variance tracking include:

- Discontinuation of supportive care devices (for example, an endotracheal tube, a nasogastric tube, or a Foley catheter)
- Initiation of rehabilitative therapy (for example, ambulation, exercises, or self-care activities)
- Initiation of patient education activities (for example, wound care or medication instruction)
- Completion of recommended referrals (for example, home health)
- Conversion of therapies (for example, a switch from parenteral to oral pain medication, from continuous intravenous fluids to saline lock, or an advancement of diet)

Frequently, the chart review used to build the initial critical path reveals recurrent events that seemingly influence a patient's ability to progress and recover. For example, a team developing a CareMap for coronary artery bypass may decide that the timing of extubating a patient is critical in preventing pulmonary complications. Similarly, the success of beginning early ambulation by the second postoperative day may be a key event in predicting the recovery of the cardiac patient. Key events usually must occur if a patient's recovery is to be uneventful.

However, if the chart review does not clearly reveal key events, the team may decide to implement a CareMap and collect all variance for a limited trial period or on a limited number of patients. During this trial period trends will likely emerge. Then it becomes essential for the team to review data regularly and make decisions about what data are essential. A deadline should be set for determining key events so that the team can perceive that its time is well spent. Three to six months should be an adequate time frame if staff using the CareMap are well prepared and if a sufficient volume of patients is placed on CareMaps.

It is important to recognize that not all variances require action. Shewhart[11] suggested that there are two types of causes for variance: a *constant system of chance* and *assignable causes*. Some variation always occurs because of the collective influence of multiple causes found regularly within every occurrence of the process.[12] For example, some patients experience more pain, testing delays result when patients are not prepared for transport, and some patients will develop fever over the course of an illness. If only common-chance causes influence variation in a system, the system is stable and thus predictable.[13] In this case, it would be unwise to react to common-chance causes for variance. Change for the sake of change is not necessarily beneficial. Too often, health care providers do just that because they mistakenly believe that a specific cause can be linked to each point of variation (and by acting on the cause they can reduce variation).[14] A well-intended change can disrupt a well-designed process such as a CareMap and not improve overall outcomes. In the case of common-chance cause, it is important to apply statistical methods to ensure that a variation has statistical significance; then it may be appropriate to revise a CareMap.

Sometimes a specific cause or set of circumstances not regularly present can influence variance. These assignable or special causes are known or can be discovered and action taken. When variation from a special cause is found, the fundamental process (in this case, the array of CareMap interventions and outcomes) should not change. Instead, action should be taken on the special cause. Critical to making any changes is assurance that frontline workers become involved in taking action. For example, after studying total hip patients placed on a CareMap, team members might recognize that patients who receive preadmission rehab training perform postoperative ambulation more successfully than those who have no early training. The team determines how changes can be made to have all patients undergo preadmission exercise training. In this case, the special cause for variation was positive.

However, as mentioned previously, variation can also be negative. For example, while monitoring the variance of thoracotomy patients, a team from a large midwestern teaching hospital recognized an increased incidence of postoperative air leaks. Patients were unable to have chest tubes discontinued and the LOS became extended. A review of patient cases revealed problems in how surgeons sutured the bronchial stump. Once corrected, the incidence of air leaks began to decline. Making a change when it is appropriate can improve outcomes without disrupting the entire process of care.

The Legal Ramifications of Variance

Frequently, physicians complain that critical paths represent cookbook medicine and thus prevent them from taking the necessary steps to intervene when a patient requires a different course of therapy. Additionally, many physicians fear that if CareMaps and variance reporting become part of patient medical records, there will be greater risk of litigation, especially when a patient's course does not follow the recommended treatment protocol. Consequently, there is reluctance on the part of physicians to make the established clinical interventions and outcomes defined in a CareMap visible to consumers.

From a legal viewpoint, the CareMap outlines a series of clinical judgments concerning recommended practice patterns of health care providers.[15] Further, it embodies practice guidelines while allowing documentation of variations in care and patient response. A CareMap prescribes minimal standards of care for all patients to ensure that essential elements of care are not forgotten. They do not preclude necessary medical interventions when patients fail to progress as predicted. Thus, the important issue is whether the use of written practice guidelines that prescribe or imply standards for proper patient care increases the incidence of malpractice suits.

Typically, when a medical case reaches the courtroom, the prosecution attempts to show that the standard of care appropriate for a client was not met. A sequence of care activities may be constructed on the basis of available medical record information to determine whether conventional standards for good medical care were achieved.

When hospitals do not utilize defined clinical guidelines, it is difficult to show what level of care was intended. In such cases, the medical record often reveals a morass of data showing the individual contributions of multiple caregivers rather than a single, coordinated plan of action. On the other hand, a CareMap provides an orderly method of analysis for medical care that will substantially aid jurors' understanding of the nature and sequence of care.[16] It also will reduce the need to rely on expert witnesses.

Thus, with the CareMap providing a clear picture of recommended clinical guidelines, variance recording shows how caregivers respond to changes in the clinical course of a patient. Such information must be shown in a courtroom when a physician or institution must justify clinical actions in the face of unpredicted events. As long as clinicians recognize and respond to changes in a patient's condition, select medically appropriate therapies, and evaluate the results of their actions, it is unlikely that a court of law will judge that negligence has occurred. A well-designed system of variance reporting supports an institution that must demonstrate the intent of therapies for a patient whose clinical course was poor.

The Clinical Use of Variance

In order for clinicians to use variance data effectively, variance charting and tracking systems must be in place. Additionally, the organization should ensure that staff are trained in using the CareMaps so that they can individualize patient care and monitor outcomes.

Variance Documentation Systems

Once the CareMap team has developed its standard of care and practice, a mechanism must be established for evaluating the tool's effectiveness. The executive steering committee should devise a system for variance collection and analysis. The following subsections describe different variance charting systems as well as a tool for tracking variance.

Charting Variance

It is most useful to have CareMap tools as part of an organization's documentation system along with variance reporting. Integrating standards of care and practice into the charting system makes it easier for caregivers to become familiarized with elements of the CareMap and to drive the clinical decisions that must be made during the course of a patient's illness. In addition, depending on the mechanism used by the organization to gather quality improvement information, having CareMaps as part of the documentation system supports a concurrent as well as retrospective evaluation approach. The model makes it easy for clinicians to review the overall care process during the patient's LOS or visit and also provides a source of valuable data for retrospective review.

The design of a CareMap also lends itself to charting by exception. In this system, a caregiver needs only document in the CareMap the interventions or outcomes that did not occur as predicted. This approach tends to minimize duplication on other chart forms. It should be noted that when assessment measures are a part of a path, organizations often choose to have data recorded on existing flow sheets rather than on the map itself. Flow sheets still provide a trending display that cannot be captured on most CareMap forms.

Using charting by exception, items at variance on the CareMap may be circled or checked depending on the charting system selected. (See figure 6-2.) When a variance occurs, the caregiver also documents on the map additional interventions needed

Figure 6-2. Care Path® for Thoracotomy

BARNES	**CARE PATH®** **500** **THORACOTOMY**	1

SERVICE	PHYSICIAN	
PRIMARY NURSE	PRIMARY NURSE	
DC DATE	ADM DATE	DATE OF SURGERY

A-8

Problem Number	PATIENT PROBLEMS / NURSING DIAGNOSES
#1	LACK OF KNOWLEDGE RELATED TO INEXPERIENCE WITH SURGERY
#2	ALTERATION IN COMFORT RELATED TO INCISION / CHEST TUBES
#3	INEFFECTIVE BREATHING PATTERN RELATED TO PAIN / DECREASED LUNG EXPANSION
#4	IMPAIRED GAS EXCHANGE RELATED TO VENTILATION - PERFUSION INEQUALITIES
#5	INEFFECTIVE AIRWAY CLEARANCE RELATED TO PAIN / INCREASED SECRETIONS
#6	POTENTIAL FOR IMPAIRED MOBILITY RELATED TO PAIN AND DISCOMFORT

#	4, 7, 10	6, 8, 9	4, 5	3, 5, 10	6
	ASSESSMENT / MONITORING	**CONSULTS**	**PROCEDURES / TEST**	**TREATMENT**	**ACTIVITY**
PRE ADMIT ADMISSION	Pre-op Workup Assess Braden Scale Assess for fall prevention	Pulmonary Rehab. Social Work Chaplain Physical Therapy Thoracic Oncology Coordinator	Identify high risk via exercise testing PFT ABG CXR PT/PTT SMA 6/12 CBC T & S UA	Appropriate bed surface for Braden Scale Enroll in fall prevention program if appropriate	
DAY DOS	A-line Telemetry Oximetry I & O $S_aO_2 \geq 90$ with or without supplemental O_2	Chaplain to check need for referral to own clergy	Foley CT to suction x2 ABG x1 x2 SMA 6 CBC CXR	O_2 Aerosols x1 x2 x3 x4 CPT x1 x2 x3 x4 by Nursing, Physical Therapy • CPT positions: _____ _____ _____ _____ • Vibration • Percussion Incentive Spirometer / TCDB q 2 hr.	Bedrest / chair Passive range of motion
DAY POD 1 OU	Weight VS q 4 hrs. x1 x2 x3 x4 x5 x6 A-line Telemetry Oximetry I & O		Foley CT to suction x2 ABG x1 SMA 6 CBC CXR	O_2 Aerosols x1 x2 x3 x4 CPT x1 x2 x3 x4 by Nursing, Physical Therapy • CPT positions: _____ _____ _____ _____ • Vibration • Percussion Incentive Spirometer / TCDB q 2 hr.	Chair x1 x2 x3 Active range of motion Ambulate as tolerated BID / with assistive device

SIGNATURE	INIT.	SIGNATURE	INIT.	SIGNATURE	INIT.

(Continued on next page)

Figure 6-2. (Continued)

| 2 |

BARNES — CARE PATH® 500 THORACOTOMY

CNS	DIETARY	RT
HOME HEALTH	OT	OTHER
PT	SW	OTHER

A-8

Problem Number	PATIENT PROBLEMS / NURSING DIAGNOSES
#7	POTENTIAL FOR DECREASED CARDIAC OUTPUT RELATED TO ALTERATION IN RHYTHM
#8	ANXIETY RELATED TO POTENTIAL CHANGE IN HEALTH STATUS
#9	SPIRITUAL DISTRESS RELATED TO IMPLICATIONS OF DIAGNOSIS AND THERAPY
#10	ALTERATION IN SKIN INTEGRITY RELATED TO SURGICAL PROCEDURE / DISEASE PROCESS

2	3, 4, 5, 6	1 - 10	1, 2, 6, 8, 9, 10	1, 8, 9	INITIALS (SEE KEY AT BOTTOM)
MEDS / IVS	NUTRITION	PATIENT / FAMILY EDUCATION	DISCHARGE PLANNING	PSYCHOSOCIAL/ EMOTIONAL/ SPIRITUAL NEEDS	
		Pre-op teaching by: Nursing, Physical Therapy Plan of care and teaching needs have been mutually set with pt./family. • Give pt. education booklet • View pt. education video • Give admission letter **Pt. able to verbalize:** - **Type of surgery/incision.** - **Pre-op preparation** - **Pain management** - **Chest tubes** - **Diet** - **Pulmonary hygiene/activity** - **Monitoring/O$_2$ Rx** **Pt. able to return - demonstrate: Incentive Spirometer/TCDB/ PCA use Pt./family verbalizes understanding of care path and family waiting area.**	**Pt. family verbalizes understanding of expected outcomes and length of stay**	Listen to pt. concerns related to diagnosis/ surgery.	
Epid. or PCA IV IV antibiotic _____	Ice chips	- Review plan of care for today and introduce plan for tomorrow.		Family supported during surgery: • timely updates • emotional/ spiritual care • collaborate with own clergy **Verbalizes feelings regarding diagnosis/ surgery Pt./family verbalizes spiritual needs and resources**	
Epid. or PCA Replace day of surgery IV site IV - Hep lock if PO intake adequate	Advance as tolerated	- Review plan of care for today and introduce plan for tomorrow.			

SIGNATURE	INIT.	SIGNATURE	INIT.	SIGNATURE	INIT.

138

Figure 6-2.   (Continued)

#	4, 7 ASSESSMENT / MONITORING	6, 8, 9 CONSULTS	4, 5 PROCEDURES / TEST	3, 5 TREATMENT	6 ACTIVITY
DAY POD 2 OU	Weight VS q 4 hrs. x1 x2 x3 x4 x5 x6 A-line Telemetry Random Oximetry with ambulation I & 0 **ABG's stable**	Check need for Social Work Consult Check need for Thoracic Oncology coordinator	~~d/c Foley~~ PA d/c 1st CT / change dressing or remove **No significant air leak / Pneumo** SMA6 CBC CXR	O$_2$ Aerosols x1 x2 x3 x4 CPT x1 x2 x3 x4 by Nursing, Physical Therapy • CPT positions: _____ _____ _____ _____ • Vibration • Percussion Incentive Spirometer / TCDB q 2 hr. *Incentive Spirometer PA* *Self use*	Chair as tolerated Ambulate BID with assistive device
DAY POD 3	Weight Check for BM _____ *AS* ~~d/c Telemetry~~ *Continue* *Telemetry* Check S$_a$O$_2$ with ambulation on room air I & 0 ~~No significant arrhythmias~~ *AS* *Conduct random* *oximetry*		d/c 2nd CT **No significant pleural effusion / pneumo** **CT drainage ≤ 50cc / shift** CXR x1 *d/c Foley PA*	O$_2$ wean with exercise d/c Aerosols CPT x1 x2 x3 x4 by Nursing, Physical Therapy • CPT positions: _____ _____ _____ _____ • Vibration • Percussion ~~Incentive Spirometer self use~~ *PA*	**Ambulate BID / with assistive device.**
DAY POD 4	Weight d/c Pulse Oximetry d/c I & 0 **Adequate I & 0** *No significant AS* *arrhythmias*	Check need for Social Work Consult Check need for Home Health	CXR x1	d/c O$_2$ **Exercise S$_a$O$_2$ ≥ 90 on room air** d/c CPT **Able to deep breath, cough and clear sputum independently**	Ambulates TID independently; d/c Physical Therapy
DAY POD 5	Weight			**CXR clear Sputum clear Lung sounds WNL**	
DAY POD 6 DISCHARGE	Weight **Weight stable** **Normal urinary / bowel function**	Check need for referral to own clergy **DC to home self care with MD / clinic follow-up**	Suture removal per MD preference **No significant infiltrate, collapse, pleural effusion or pneumothorax** **Wound clean and dry**	 **Exercise S$_a$O$_2$ ≥ 85 on room air with rest and exercise program** **CXR clear Sputum clear Lung sounds WNL**	d/c pt. **Able to perform home exercise program**

SIGNATURE	INIT.	SIGNATURE	INIT.	SIGNATURE	INIT.
Pat Adams	*PA*				
Art W. Smith	*AS*				

(Continued on next page)

Figure 6-2.   (Continued)

2	3, 4, 5, 6	1 - 9	1, 2, 6, 8, 9	1, 8, 9	INITIALS (SEE KEY AT BOTTOM)		
MEDS / IVS	NUTRITION	PATIENT / FAMILY EDUCATION	DISCHARGE PLANNING	PSYCHOSOCIAL/ EMOTIONAL/ SPIRITUAL NEEDS			
Epid. or PCA IV for PCA	**Tolerating PO fluids** *Increase fluids to 2000cc daily PA*	Review plan of care for today and introduce plan for tomorrow.			*PA*		
d/c Epid. or PCA d/c IV Start PO pain meds Dulcolax/Laxative if no BM	**Good PO intake** *Increase fluids to 2000cc daily PA*	Teach self care and self ambulation Teach chest mobility Review plan of care for today and introduce plan for tomorrow **Pt. able to demonstrate self care** **Pt. able to demonstrate chest mobility**	Arrange outpatient oncology referrals if needed		*AS*		
Pain controlled with oral analgesics		Teach strength/flexibility exercises Review plan of care for today and introduce plan for tomorrow - Begin review of discharge instructions in pt. education booklet. • Wound care • Diet • Activity • Medications • Comfort measures • When to call MD **Pt. able to demonstrate strength/ flexibility exercises**	Arrange outpatient pulmonary rehab. if needed Check need for transportation/home equipment, etc.	Help pt. identify resources at DC: ie support groups, Cancer Information Center, ALA, ACS, etc.	*AS*		
		Teach home exercises and give activity log Continue discharge teaching Review plan of care for today and introduce plan for tomorrow Check smoking cessation needs for resources (ALA, ACS) **Pt. able to demonstrate home exercise and use of activity log**					
IV sites without phlebitis Afebrile Pain free or pain controlled with oral analgesics	Good PO intake	Review DC teaching, activity, medications, self care, wound care, diet, comfort measures. - Review plan of care for today and introduce plan for tomorrow Arrange MD follow-up Review Oncology needs and education resources (ACS, CIC) **Pt. verbalizes understanding of DC instructions.** **Able to function independently in ADLs and self care** **Verbalizes understanding of oncology status and follow-up**	Demonstrates/ verbalizes under-standing of care needs	Able to express feelings about beliefs, values and meaning in relation to current health status.			
SIGNATURE	INIT.	SIGNATURE	INIT.	SIGNATURE		INIT.	

to reverse a negative variance, to reschedule an outcome that remains unmet, or to list interventions or outcomes met earlier than predicted. The caregiver must demonstrate when new interventions are planned to accommodate for any variance that alters patient progress. Figure 6-2 illustrates an example of a patient undergoing a thoracotomy. In this case, the patient fails to have a Foley catheter discontinued on postop day (POD) 2. The nurse circles the variance "d/c Foley" and moves the intervention to POD 3. Similarly, the nurse adds "increase fluid intake to 2000 cc daily" to the interventions for PODs 2 and 3.

In another example, the outcome "incentive spirometer self-use" is moved to POD 2. The patient has achieved an outcome earlier than predicted. The nurse circles the outcome on POD 3 as a variance and enters the outcome under treatment measures for POD 2. With the patient showing progress in using the incentive spirometer, the health care team will look for opportunities to further support self-care. The possibility arises that the patient will be receptive to more education at an earlier stage.

Tracking Variance

Unless the organization has CareMaps computerized, variance will need to be recorded on a tracking form that can later be used for variance analysis and CQI activities. A variance tracking form should include columns for the date, the description of the variance, the type of variance (source), the action taken, and the caregiver's signature. (See figure 6-3.) Additional columns can be used to record the CareMap number, whether the variance was an outcome, or the related patient problem at variance. Again, it is each organization's decision to determine how much detail is needed when recording variance. In the example given earlier, the thoracotomy patient experienced a variance involving a delay in discontinuing the Foley catheter. On the variance tracking form, the nurse identifies the day and time, lists the variance "d/c Foley," and lists the action to be taken: "d/c Foley on POD 3 after increasing fluids, if urine output greater than 1000 cc." In addition, the variance form shows that the outcome—"incentive spirometer self-use"—was achieved one day early.

When the CareMap is a part of the documentation system, typically the variance tracking form also will be placed in the medical record. Many organizations have created a two-part form so that a copy can be sent to the appropriate individual or department analyzing variance trends. Additionally, when a patient condition causes a variance, many organizations require a progress note to ensure meaningful, focused documentation. Narrative notes written in SOAP, PIE, or a focused charting format allow clinicians to communicate any details about the patient's condition that warrant continued intervention.

Educational Support

When CareMaps are first implemented, the project manager or case manager must provide the educational support necessary to assist staff in assigning patients appropriately to maps and in using the maps to individualize patient care. Ultimately, the clinicians must be accountable for patient outcomes on the CareMaps.

Assigning Accountability

Assignment of accountability will vary depending on the delivery of care method employed. In the case of primary nursing, for example, one registered nurse takes ownership for coordinating the patient's nursing care and ensuring that other disciplines become involved as outlined on the map. He or she is proactive and uses the CareMap to keep priorities in focus. On the other hand, in the case of team or functional nursing, no one nurse is accountable to the patient. Although the nurse manager has accountability, he or she also has other responsibilities. Thus, accountability often

Patricia Potter

Figure 6-3. Care Path® Variance Tracking Form

BARNES

Care Path® Variance Tracking Form

Care Path® Number _410_   **Division** _5100_
Entered in CRT: Date _5/7_   **Initial** _____

ADDRESSOGRAPH

√ If Outcome

DATE	TIME	CARE PATH DAY	VARIANCE	√	REASON	ACTION PLAN	INITIAL
5/9	1620	POD2	Foley D/C		Urine output 600cc	D/C Foley on POD3 if	
					for 24 hours	urine output 1000cc	
5/9	1800	POD2	Incentive spiro-		Patient performs		
			meter self use		IS well, indepen-		
					dently, initiates		
					breathing exercise		
5/10	0830	POD3	Arrythmia (A fib)		Arrythmia may	Continue telemetry	
					be related to poor	Conduct random oximetry	
					medication control		

Signature/Initials

140970 Revised 1/93

142

defaults to the physician.[17] In the functional or team model, the physician is unable to give attention to the details involved in the coordination of patient care.

Zander refers to a care management model in which there is structuring of accountability for client outcomes at the care delivery level.[18] With care management typically one caregiver coordinates care from admission through discharge within an acute care setting. A single multidisciplinary plan, such as a CareMap, ensures all caregivers work with one plan. Numerous hospitals have begun to assign registered nurses in care manager or coordinator roles. These staff work in collaboration with other nursing staff to manage either distinct patient populations, patients located on a single nursing unit, or patients managed by a single physician. As a care coordinator, the nurse may give patient care or ultimately serve as a case manager during the acute episode of illness.

In case management, a single caregiver manages the clients' care across a continuum. Care is coordinated across nursing units and between agencies. Clients requiring case management are high risk and usually experiencing complicated problems.

Learning to Use Variance to Individualize Care

With the CareMap system, variances become more visible than in less-structured clinical methods.[19] Because it becomes obvious when a patient's course is sidetracked, clinicians must learn to use this information in a proactive way to take corrective action. Project managers should develop an environment for caregivers to learn from variance so that clinical decision-making skills are strengthened. It is even more desirable when members of different disciplines collaborate to analyze variances and choose the best approaches to care.

When a caregiver manages a patient on a CareMap, the tool requires that several questions be answered. These include:[20]

- What interventions should be delivered by the staff and how should the patient and family respond?
- What actually is happening; is there a variance?
- What is causing the variance?
- What action must the caregiver take?

During each change of shift report and any multidisciplinary conference, clinicians review patient progress on the path and note the next series of interventions for which they are responsible. Depending on the variance, the CareMap lets caregivers know what direction to take in patient care. If variance occurs, it is not in isolation with all other activities. A caregiver can quickly assess the extent to which a variance may influence other interventions or outcomes. For example, if the thoracotomy patient were to develop significant arrhythmias, contrary to the outcome predicted on POD 3 (figure 6-2, p. 137), the nurse would likely continue telemetry and then make a determination as to the patient's activity plan. Perhaps the nurse would return to interventions used on POD 2 and measure random oximetry more frequently. The occurrence of variance takes place in the context of the patient's total clinical plan. Judgments are enhanced as caregivers identify problems earlier, take action within the context of the patient's clinical needs, and evaluate the success of interventions.

Sometimes a patient is at variance for a prolonged period of time. In this case, members of the health care team must gather to decide if the CareMap remains a useful tool in planning care. If the necessary interventions are no longer reflective of what is represented on a CareMap, the team may decide to discontinue its use. An example might be a patient who experiences a stroke following a coronary artery bypass. The clinical interventions prescribed for treatment of the stroke are not normally incorporated into a standard CareMap for coronary artery bypass. If an institution has developed multiple CareMaps, the team has a different option. It can decide to place the patient on a new map—in this case, cerebrovascular accident.

Clinical decision making is a skill that develops over time. When staff are relatively new to their roles, it is helpful for project managers to use CareMaps as teaching tools. The learning environment should be supportive, and periodic monitoring with one-to-one interaction with caregivers reinforces the value of CareMaps in the overall process of patient care. For example, a reviewer can ask why a particular intervention was delayed, what the intent of the physician was who ordered an additional test, or how the caregiver has planned to adjust interventions so that a delayed outcome can be met. Variances from the CareMap should be looked on as opportunities to focus on the evaluation of patient progress so that adjustments can be made to promote patient recovery. This level of interaction also helps to focus on the accountability of each clinician for individualizing patient care.

Retrospective Use of Variance for Quality Improvement

The clinical decision making generated from use of a CareMap is a simple application of the scientific method (nursing process). Caregivers routinely assess the patient's status on the map, plan on the basis of collaboratively determined outcome measures, intervene, and evaluate variance so as to analyze the patient's status.[21] Over time, as more patients are cared for using a CareMap, clinicians begin to evaluate the effects of care for groups of patients. Team members analyze aggregate variance to ensure continuous quality improvement.

Choosing a Format for Reporting Variance Data

Before a team can retrospectively review CareMaps, data must be made available in a concise and meaningful format. The hospital must decide who will extract data from variance tracking forms and how the data will be displayed for review. Typically, hospitals use their quality improvement and/or utilization review staff to collate and record data. After a patient is discharged, variance forms are removed from the medical chart and sent to the appropriate department. In some instances, project managers themselves report data, although this can be very time-consuming and distract them from the important work of managing patient care.

When recording variance, many hospitals have found it useful to identify it by source. (See figure 6-4.) The broad variance categories enable the clinicians evaluating CareMaps to see if there are recurrent trends in the types of variance that occur. This

Figure 6-4.   Variance Source Codes

A	Patient/Family	1 Condition
		2 Decision
		3 Availability
		4 Other
B	Clinician	5 Order
		6 Decision
		7 Response Time
		8 Other
C	Hospital	9 Bed/Appointment Availability
		10 Information/Data Availability
		11 Other
D	Community	12 Placement/Home Care
		13 Transportation
		14 Other

form of analysis can help to identify quality improvement opportunities in areas such as system delivery of services, clinician response time, and preventive clinical measures. It must be remembered that when variance recording is part of the documentation system, caregivers must record all clinical variances. However, the CareMap team will likely decide not to formally report all variances for retrospective review. In the example of the thoracotomy patient, the postponement of discontinuing the Foley catheter was a patient variance resulting from his or her condition. This type of variance is unlikely to become a pattern over time. The postponement of discontinuing the Foley was a common cause for variance and does not warrant formal review.

Another system for reporting variance is by using the categories of care (assessments, tests, activity, discharge planning, and so on) that comprise the CareMap. If data collectors can enter variance information into a computer database, types of variance can easily be sorted for review to determine whether the occurrence of different types of variances warrants action. (See figure 6-5.) Depending on how variances are coded by staff during documentation, trending reports can sort by positive and negative variance.[22] (See figure 6-6.)

Project managers and the CareMap team analyze variance, the time frames within which it occurs, and the corresponding actions taken by clinicians to determine if changes need to be made in the approach to care. The evaluation of significant variance over time allows caregivers to identify potential causes for patient characteristics (for example, complications), care processes (for example, pain management), and resources (for example, lab tests) that produced observed outcomes. Ideally, the CareMap team wants to use information and knowledge gained from monitoring variance to achieve optimal patient outcomes through improved clinical decision making and service delivery.[23] This is called *outcomes management*. The team may identify the need to improve the processes of care already identified on the CareMap, revise the map itself, or make improvements in the operational systems affecting its use. (See figure 6-7.) When the team commits to monitoring only variances from 100 percent of

Figure 6-5. Variance Report by Category of Care

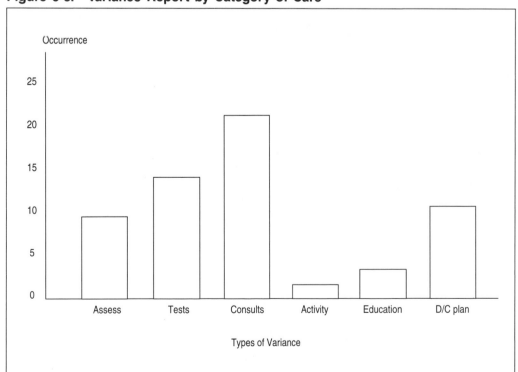

intermediate goals and outcomes and 100 percent of key tasks, trending of variance becomes more meaningful. In addition, this decision minimizes the chances of the team spending too much time analyzing common causes for variance.

Regardless of how refined a variance reporting system may be, invariably CareMap team members will need to look at patient records to critically review variance trends. For example, in a case where 8 out of 40 total hip patients develop a hip dislocation following surgery, the incidence of hip dislocation alone will not allow a team to expose the processes of care that contributed to the complication. Although intuitively staff members may know what causes repeated complications, detailed chart reviews for

Figure 6-6. Positive/Negative Variance Comparison Report

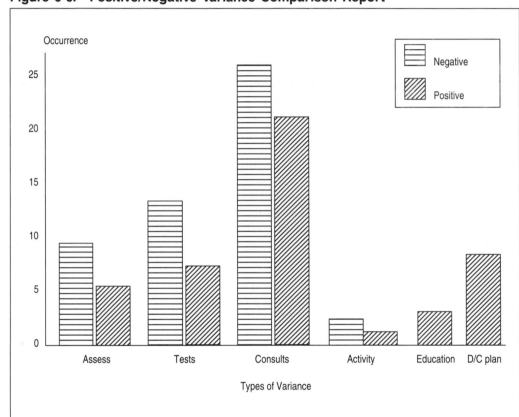

Figure 6-7. CareMap Improvement Opportunities

Improve Processes of Care	• Improve promptness of consults • Provide educational materials to educational plan • Initiate team discussions at critical points in patient's recovery • Involve patient and family more directly in monitoring progress on CareMap
Revise CareMap	• Delete or add tests, procedures, or treatments • Revise time frames for outcome achievement • Revise time frames for interventions • Change frequency of interventions
Change Operational Systems	• Revise admission process or discharge process • Change medication delivery system • Introduce new discipline into the collaborative plan • Develop better patient transport system • Initiate preadmit therapies

cases of variance will greatly assist them in building a clear clinical picture as to what went wrong. If CareMaps are built into an automated charting system, it can become easier to retrieve relevant clinical information for review.

Providing Feedback to Clinicians

Integral to any CQI effort is a provision for feedback to clinicians using the CareMaps. Depending on how an organization structures its quality improvement program, a mechanism must be in place to ensure that clinicians receive useful, meaningful, and accurate data to help modify the care process. Any successful quality improvement effort must become part of the staff's daily work. Staff familiar with a system's strengths and weaknesses are in the best position to interpret data and know when there are opportunities to improve. Similarly, if a team of clinicians makes recommendations for system changes, it is the responsibility of the organization to carry them through. The Joint Commission on Accreditation of Healthcare Organizations requires hospitals to provide the necessary resources when performance improvement opportunities are identified.[24]

Conclusion

CareMaps are not an end in themselves. The process of patient care is dynamic and changes with individual patient characteristics and caregiver skills and judgments. Variance is the one clinical approach that, when used concurrently, guarantees a comprehensive and collaborative approach to managing patient problems. Variance analysis forces evaluation. Clinicians become accountable for the outcomes of their care, learning to inquire as to what interventions create the best results. Once a health care team learns to respond to variance appropriately, patient outcomes are enhanced.

A CareMap is a tool to improve the daily course of clinical work. In order for meaningful changes to occur retrospectively, a team must not merely take action as individual variances occur but also must look at the collective of patients managed on a single CareMap and ask whether the process and systems of care are complementary and function optimally. Variance trending helps caregivers understand the need for change, take action, reevaluate the results, and maintain improvement.

References

1. Nash, D. B. Accountability for hospital quality: the role of clinical practice guidelines. *Joint Commission Journal on Quality Improvement* 19(9):396–400, 1993.

2. Davies, A. R., and others. Outcomes assessment in clinical settings: a consensus statement on principles and best practices in project management. *Joint Commission Journal on Quality Improvement* 20(1):6–16, 1994.

3. Zander, K. Physicians, CareMaps, and collaboration. *The New Definition* 7(1):1–4, Winter 1992.

4. Zander, K. Quantifying, managing, and improving quality, part I: how CareMaps link CQI to the patient. *The New Definition* 7(2):1–4, Spring 1992.

5. Nash.

6. Batalden, P. B., and Stoltz, P. K. A framework for the continual improvement of health care: building and applying professional and improvement knowledge to test changes in daily work. *Joint Commission Journal on Quality Improvement* 19(10):424–47, 1993.

7. Zander, K. Quantifying, managing, and improving quality, part III: using variance concurrently. *The New Definition* 7(4):1–4, Fall 1992.

8. Batalden and Stoltz.

9. Health Care Advisory Board. Special Research: Second Generation Lessons on Critical Care Paths. Report to the annual membership. Washington, DC: Health Care Advisory Board, Spring 1993.

10. Zander, Fall 1992.

11. Shewhart, W. A. *The Economic Control of Quality of the Manufactured Product.* New York City: Van Nostrand, 1931; reprinted Milwaukee: ASQC Quality Press, 1980.

12. Batalden and Stoltz.

13. Batalden and Stoltz.

14. Batalden and Stoltz.

15. Nolin, C. E., and Lang, C. G. *An Analysis of the Use and Effect of CareMap Tools in Medical Malpractice Litigation.* Expert Library Vol. 1. South Natick, MA: The Center for Case Management, 1994.

16. Nolin and Lang.

17. Zander, K. Responsive restructuring, part IV: care management and case management. *The New Definition* 9(2):1-4, Spring 1994.

18. Zander, Spring 1994.

19. Zander, Fall 1992.

20. Zander, Fall 1992.

21. Zander, Fall 1992.

22. Hofmann, P. Critical path method: an important tool for coordinating clinical care. *Joint Commission Journal on Quality Improvement* 19(7):235-46, 1993.

23. Davies and others.

24. Joint Commission on Accreditation of Healthcare Organizations. *1994 Accreditation Manual for Hospitals.* Chicago: Oakbrook Terrace, IL: JCAHO, 1994.

CHAPTER SEVEN

Integration of CareMap Tools into the Documentation System

Maria Hill

The adequacy of documentation of care delivery and the mechanisms in place to provide documentation have been frequent themes in the medical records, hospital risk management, and nursing literature for the past three decades. Three major issues have been identified: (1) the amount of information to be recorded, (2) the lack of a consistent structure in which to record the information, and (3) the number and variety of forms and/or computer entries required to record the information. These issues all contribute to the time-consuming nature of the documentation process, accounting for approximately one-third of a professional practitioner's time. With the implementation and evolution of the CareMap system, these issues are forcing CareMap project managers to consider how to expand the tool to include care documentation.

This chapter describes principles that can be used to make the CareMap tool the core of the medical record and documentation system. It discusses issues regarding the current documentation system, describes the characteristics of a fully automated system, and suggests a review of patient education in the CareMap concept.

The Current Documentation System

In an examination of current documentation systems, most CareMap design teams find a plethora of documentation forms and chart notation formats. These include:

- Quantitative entries on clinical data flow sheets
- Physician orders
- Incident report forms
- Medical treatment records and qualitative entries on the nursing Kardex™
- Medical and routine progress notes

Additionally, information is often replicated in multiple places and replicated inconsistently. Much of the information is repeated within and across services, adding significantly to rework performed by multiple professionals. Finally, when separate sections exist for each discipline's progress notations, the patient's written history often is disjointed and difficult to review. Generally, team members are awestruck by the magnitude of the issue faced and appreciate the structure, continuity, and consistency offered by the multidisciplinary CareMap tool when it is made the core of the medical record.

Integration of CareMap Tools into the Documentation System

When the CareMap tool is used only as a guide for care, rather than as both a plan and document of care delivered (that is, as a permanent part of the medical record), it is used inconsistently to manage the care rendered. Likewise, when the CareMap tool is added to the cumbersome, labor-intensive documentation system without replacing other forms, its use dramatically declines. Therefore, to make the system accurate, concise, and user-friendly, as well as to decrease the amount of written rework required of staff, project managers are searching for methods to integrate CareMap and variance tools into existing hospital documentation and information/data management systems. At the same time, project managers are struggling with the amount of detail that can be placed on the CareMap tool and the documents the tool can easily replace. In other words, it is a challenge to determine the level at which the CareMap tool be integrated into the current documentation system.

To embark on this process, it is imperative to consider the purposes of the medical record. According to the Joint Commission on Accreditation of Healthcare Organizations[1] and Pozgar,[2] the medical record has the following purposes:

- To provide a basis for planning patient care
- To record the course of a patient's illness and changing condition
- To record the patient's course of treatment
- To furnish communication between the practitioners responsible for and/or contributing to the patient's care
- To serve as a database for statistical reporting, evaluation, continuing education, and research
- To assist in protecting the legal interests of the patient, the hospital, and the practitioners
- To furnish information necessary for third-party billing

The CareMap system provides a strong core for the medical record and can serve as both the plan and record of care for two obvious reasons:

1. It integrates key issues identified in the JCAHO's Agenda for Change initiative (figure 5-10, p. 128), including a focus on interdisciplinary team management of patients, patient care outcomes over methods, functionally grouped standards, patient and family education, and information management.
2. It well reflects the work required to move a patient case type along a continuum of care toward outcomes.

It is logical to build the documentation system on a well-constructed tool that organizes the health care team; prioritizes the problems, issues, and needs of a patient case type; and reflects the intermediate goals and outcomes to be achieved.

Documentation entry on a CareMap tool can provide a number of benefits. These include:

- An interdisciplinary planning tool and document of collaborative care communications
- An accurate representation of the course of treatment, changes in condition, and care rendered for the case type
- Intermediate goals and discharge outcomes achieved

- A database for statistical reporting through variance analysis (continuous quality improvement) and exception charting
- A format for conducting applied research

However, it is important to note that the CareMap tool cannot be the entire documentation system, nor can it be a quick fix to poor clinician documentation resulting from inadequate understanding of the elements to be charted; sloppy, inconsistent practice; and/or failure to take the time to either document elements or comply with standards.

Designing a CareMap Documentation Format

To accomplish integration of the CareMap tool into the documentation system, three steps need to be taken. These are:

1. The project manager should assemble a team to design a format to meet the organization's needs. The design team should include members representing different disciplines including nursing management and staff; social service; pharmacy; physical, occupational, and speech therapy; nutrition; utilization and quality management; medical records; information systems; and education/training. Membership also should include key individuals assigned to documentation issues. A chair should be appointed, a meeting schedule established, educational sessions provided on the CareMap system, and the team charge identified.
2. The team should then review the current documentation system by collecting documentation forms, process-flowcharting the current system, and identifying the system's strengths and limitations compared to the identified desired functions brainstormed and prioritized by the team.
3. The team also should investigate the requirements of the institution through existing policies and procedures and state and federal regulating agencies.

The design team also must address other factors in its design considerations, including goals and functions of the format; functional format, layout, and tool location; and interventional categories.

Goals and Functions

When a CareMap format is designed to incorporate documentation, the goals and functions to be achieved should be outlined. For example, the format should:

- Accommodate a multidisciplinary record of care
- Be logical and intuitive in organization
- Be user-friendly
- Be designed in a grid and cell format as a precursor to a computerized spreadsheet
- Meet regulatory requirements of medical records
- Incorporate legal considerations

Functional Format, Layout, and Tool Location

Functional format, layout, and tool location are issues that also must be considered when designing a CareMap documentation format. The functional format of a well-designed CareMap tool contains a number of elements. These include:

- A section for general patient information
- An index of problems or issues associated with the case type
- Intermediate goals and discharge outcomes associated with the case type
- A critical path that is a cause-and-effect grid of multidisciplinary interventions designed to move the patient toward the desired outcomes within an estimated period of time
- A time line with benchmarks that indicate clinical progression stated in hours/ days/weeks/clinical phases/visits and which is applicable to the interventions, intermediate goals, and discharge outcomes
- A variance analysis sheet

Layout and tool location issues requiring discussion include:

- Placement of addressograph and patient identification on every page
- Identification of allergies
- Placement of the tool in the medical record for ease of retrieval of information and duplication
- Layout options available and their pros and cons (for example, landscape, portrait, booklet, poster, accordion, and trifold displays)

These issues are dependent on current layout and methods used to store the medical record.

Interventional Categories

The team also must discuss the interventional categories that will exist within the grid, the definitions of these categories, and an identification process for the professionals responsible for direct care within each of these categories. Following are the key interventional categories in the traditional critical path:

- Diagnostic studies
- Consults
- Diet
- Activity
- Medications
- Treatments
- Discharge planning
- Patient/family education

Additional categories used by several institutions include assessments, psychosocial, and equipment and supplies.

The design team should provide definitions for each category because an intervention may appropriately fall into two categories. For example, the administration of oxygen can be considered both a treatment and a medication. The team must define in which category this intervention will be consistently placed in all CareMap tools developed in the institution. Doing so will reinforce consistency across case types in terms of language, approach to patient care, and clinician use.

Transforming Traditional Documentation Formats

As mentioned previously, the completed CareMap tool is created by a talented team of experts. Its content includes the typical interventions to be completed and intermediate goals and discharge outcomes to be realized by 60 to 80 percent of the patients cared for within a specific case type. In the medical record, the information and data are typically captured in physician orders, standards of care, and medical and routine progress notes written by various professionals. When the CareMap tool is approved as a part of the medical record, components of documents can be revamped. For example, the medical and routine progress notations would focus on the lack of patient progress with regard to anticipated intermediate goals and outcomes as outlined in the CareMap tool. Thus, the traditional progress note would be transformed into a lack of progress or exception note.

The traditional formats used to structure notes written in the progress note section can be easily adapted to this philosophy of documentation. The SOAP (subjective, objective, assessment and plan), PIE (problem, intervention, evaluation), or focused charting format will now reflect the problem, issue, or variance that has arisen and the plan to deal with it.

Issues for future development in CareMap tool documentation include:

- All disciplines providing direct care documentation on the signature log
- Charting by exception format from standards adopted by the entire multidisciplinary team
- Integrating interdisciplinary assessment and discharge planning tool to complement the CareMap tool

Addressing Key Questions

Integration of a CareMap tool into a documentation system raises a number of questions. Following is a list of the most common questions and responses:

- *Is this a document of nursing interventions?* Yes, routine nursing interventions are preprinted and located in the assessment, treatment, activity, diet, discharge planning, and patient education sections.
- *Is this a multidisciplinary document of interventions?* Yes, these tools are created by appropriate members of the multidisciplinary team. Outlined and sequenced within the appropriate sections of the CareMap tool are the usual interventions performed for particular groups of patients.
- *Will transcription of physician orders be incorporated into the tool?* Yes, standing orders and/or general patterns of orders are preprinted on the map. In addition, written, individualized orders can be transcribed onto the appropriate categories.
- *What documents will this tool incorporate, reducing the number of forms?* Condensed into the tool are independent discipline plans of care, the traditional nursing Kardex™, normal patient progress identified by interventions, intermediate goals, and discharge outcomes. In addition, depending on the degree to which the team decides to integrate the tool, patient education records and discharge planning or instruction forms can be incorporated. Some institutions have included a statement and signature line for patients indicating review and agreement with the critical pathway. However, the tool cannot substitute and incorporate an initial database and assessment; include information written on flow sheets (for example, vital signs, weights, lab values, and assessment results); and so on. When efforts are made to make the CareMap tool the entire documentation system, its focus gets lost in the minutiae and it becomes difficult to track the patient's clinical progress through the plan of care. It also becomes difficult to track the patient's ability to meet intermediate goals and outcomes.
- *Where will the tool be located on the unit?* It often is located either at the patient's bedside or in a sleeve in the front of the medical record. The key issue is to make it accessible to all practitioners. Collaborative use is essential and difficult to realize using a paper trail system. Institutions that place the tool

in a Kardex™ holder find that it is rarely used by disciplines other than nursing.

- *How will the plan be individualized to the patient, and where will the information be located on the tool?* When used for shift-to-shift management of the patient, information related to his or her condition and needs can be added into each cell category. The CareMap is a dynamic tool that requires appropriate updating of the problem list, intermediate goals, outcomes, and interventions. Information also should be captured on the variance sheet for aggregate tracking and monitoring purposes. A "lack of progress note" may be written to communicate in detail the problem identified, the action plan, and the outcome to be realized for problem or issue resolution.

- *How will the disciplines responsible for signing off interventions and outcomes be indicated?* They could be identified on the CareMap tool, as has been done in the case of an orthopedic CareMap tool created at Lovelace Medical Center in Albuquerque, New Mexico. (See figure 7-1.) This makes clear who has ultimate accountability for specific outcomes of care. At times, two disciplines will share responsibility. For example, both nurses and respiratory therapists can sign off interventions and outcomes to promote patient learning about proper techniques for coughing, deep breathing, and use of incentive spirometry pre- and postoperatively. In addition to clarifying the responsibilities of each discipline for the care of the patient, this approach organizes the team to ensure that identified interventions and outcomes are met for each patient, decreases the amount of rework performed by different practitioners, and provides a mechanism to track individual accountability when the system fails.

- *Will this reflect a shift-by-shift and/or 24-hour period division of labor?* Typically, standard templates are created in one of two formats. One format displays two signature columns behind each time interval. (See figure 7-2, p. 156.) (Figure 7-3, p. 157, shows that this same format can be accomplished through use of a separate sheet with a signature log.) These columns represent night, day, and evening shifts. The advantage to this format is that staff can sign off each individual intervention and outcome in the appropriate time interval, which enhances each practitioner's accountability for each intervention and outcome. The disadvantage is that this format takes up more space and thus reduces the number of time intervals that can be displayed on a piece of paper, reducing the visual display of the episode of care. This may inhibit the practitioner's ability to change focus from a shift to an episode of care for the patient and family.

  The second format displays a set of signature columns at the end of a 24-hour time frame. (See figure 7-4, p. 158.) The advantage to this format is that the clinician can view greater time intervals within the continuum of care. The disadvantage is that it is less clear who completed which individual interventions and outcomes.

- *Can all care elements requiring documentation be built into a CareMap tool?* This question is still being debated. For more simplistic, ambulatory case types, it may be plausible to build more components requiring documentation into the CareMap tool. For example, the assessment parameters and quantitative data may be recorded onto the tool. However, for complex case types it appears impossible to absorb all these data elements onto a two-dimensional paper tool without causing chaos and loss of the visual display of the patient's clinical progression to end outcomes through the episode of illness.

- *What should the system look like for patients whose care is not guided by a CareMap tool? Can the hospital support two different documentation systems? At what point has critical mass been reached to change the entire system over to CareMap tools?* Four choices exist regarding integration of the CareMap tool into the documentation system:

Figure 7-1.   Total Knee CareMap Document (Excerpt)

Day 4 (POD 3)	N	D	E
Nurse/RT Patient demonstrates proper techniques for C&DB and use of IS.			
Nurse Patient understands use of CPM (if ordered).			
CM Patient recalls knee precautions.			
PT Patient demonstrates proper weight-bearing status, ROM (if applicable), and understands TKR precautions.			
Dietitian Patient demonstrates good comprehension of coumadin diet.			
CM/Nurse Patient/family know discharge plans.			

Key:

- RT = Respiratory Therapist
- C&DB = Coughing and Deep Breathing
- IS = Incentive Spirometry
- CPM = Continuous Passive Motion Machine
- CM = Case Manager
- ROM = Range of Motion
- TKR = Total Knee Replacement

Reprinted, with permission, from Lovelace Medical Center, Albuquerque, New Mexico.

Figure 7-2. Illustration of Signature Log and Initial Column Tied to Date Columns

	Signature Log (A complete signature must be entered under the correlating time column when initialed entries are made in the CareMap Tool.)			
Date				
	Signature	**Int.**	**Signature**	**Int.**
Consults				
Dietitian				
Physician				
PT/OT/Rehab				
N u r s i n g				
R e s p				
Social Worker				
Other				
Other				
Other				
Other				
CareMap Authors:				

—The tool is approved as a stand-alone document and permanent part of the medical record, and replaces only the disciplines' independent plans of care.

—It is partially integrated into the documentation system, replacing the individual disciplines' plans of care, portions of the nursing Kardex™, and normal progress notes.

—It is completely integrated into the documentation system and a multitude of documents are reconstructed using it as the core of the medical record.

—All patient care is recorded on a CareMap tool format, with the use of blank tools for undeveloped diagnoses.

The key to successful implementation of the last two options lies within the percentage of patients managed on preprinted CareMap tools. The more dramatically the documentation system is changed to accommodate the CareMap tool as the core of the medical record, the more dramatically the other processes are affected. For example, before eliminating the traditional nursing Kardox™, the design team should query how it is used by the unit secretary, the nursing assistant, and consulting services to complete required work. Then the team should determine how to most simplistically perform that work within the structure of the newly created documentation system. Thus, it is essential to ensure that a critical mass of CareMap tools is being used to guide patient care prior to revamping the entire documentation system.

- *What are the legal implications of this new documentation system?* Often professional staff, most notably physicians and nurses, voice concerns when project managers discuss development and implementation of CareMap tools and variance/exception charting. Generally, these staff are concerned about the use of written guidelines prescribing standards for patient care, the potential need to deviate from the guidelines to meet individual patient needs, and the impact of the notion "if it isn't documented, it wasn't done" on the incidence of malpractice suits. In response to these concerns, Nolin and Lang[3] write that the use of practice standards does not create significant new risks and actually may reduce the risk and cost of litigation. In addition, when the CareMap tool is approved as a permanent part of the medical record, when signatures following completion of interventions and outcomes are entered, and when variances are identified and documented as a lack of progress with concomitant identification of plans to deal with them, it is likely that stronger documentation is in place than the documentation consistently recorded in the previous system. Casebooks are filled with examples showing poor record keeping and conflictual

Figure 7-3. Illustration of Signature Tied to Initialed Date Columns on Separate Page from the Map

Signature Log		
Date		
	Day 4 **Floor**	**Day 5** **Floor**
Consults:		
Dietary:		
PT/OT/Rehabilitation		
Physician		
Night		
RN: Day		
Evening		
Night		
RT: Day		
Evening		
Social Worker		
Other:		
Other:		
Other:		

Figure 7-4. Illustration of Signature Log at Base of Intervention Columns

Problems/Focus	Day 1	Day 2	Day 3	Day 4	Discharge Day Day 5
1.					
2.					
3.					
Assessments					
Tests					
Treatments					
Medications					
Nutrition					
Safety/Activity					
Teaching					
Discharge Planning					
Signature Log					

professional notes as sources of liability. The CareMap will aid in defense because it is a complete plan, encourages clear communication, and enhances uniform record keeping.

- *For what areas of the CareMap tool is professional staff accountable? Paraprofessional staff?* According to the state professional practice act, health care professional staff are accountable for the overall assessment of care. Thus, it is their responsibility to review and document the problem/issue list, evaluate the plan with outlined interventions and outcomes of care, monitor the plan, and evaluate its effectiveness. Paraprofessional staff can sign off the activities or interventions they complete, such as information outlined within the treatment, diet, activity, and discharge planning sections. However, ultimately their work is the responsibility of the professional staff.

CareMap Automation

Practitioners are carefully scrutinizing how to best document care delivered in the most efficient and effective manner. Many have concluded that CareMap tools and variance management systems must not only be computerized but also must be integrated with cost accounting systems, acuity, admissions, transfer and discharge programs, order entry, utilization and quality management, materials ordering, and so on. Additionally, they believe that CareMap tools and variance management systems must span the traditional geographic boundaries of the acute, ambulatory, and community settings. As far as these clinicians are concerned, managing the continuum of health care and meeting patient/family, employer, insurer, and government demands will not be truly successful until the CareMap tool is automated and integrated with other computerized functions. At present, there are two principal barriers to integration of the CareMap system with existing information systems – either the hospital has no existing information system or the hospital's current system cannot yet support the use of CareMap tools.

Advantages to CareMap Tool Automation

There are distinct advantages to integrating CareMap tools into the documentation system through automation.[4] These advantages include the following:

- *It creates a three-dimensional, interactive medical record and information system.* Because the manual system permits construction of only a two-dimensional paper system, users are unable to integrate the library of information stored in flow sheet graphics, policy and procedure manuals, the drug formulary, procedure preparations for patients, cost accounts, variance records, and so on. When automated and linked to these other systems through a windows application, clinicians will be able to use the computer to assist in assimilation of data that will enable them to make prudent, accurate, and timely decisions about patient care. For example, when a COPD patient presents with symptoms of pneumonia confirmed by chest X ray and sputum specimen, through the computer the physician should be able to access in real time the chest X ray and lab results, identify the organism and drugs it is sensitive to, and call up the drug formulary to determine the most effective antibiotic at the most reasonable cost.
- *It increases accessibility, with the tool being available to multiple providers in multiple geographic locations in real time.* For example, it enables the nurse to make entries at the patient bedside as care is delivered, the surgeon to view the hospitalized patient's plan of care from the surgical suite, and the home care nurse to view the patient's progress from the home care office. The current paper trail system does not allow information to be readily available to multiple providers either within or outside the acute or home care settings, and negatively affects the clinician's ability to make immediate, efficient, and effective decisions regarding patient care.
- *It enables clinicians to integrate two or more paper CareMap tools into one document to direct care for complex patients with three or more active diagnoses.* For example, it allows for ready update of CareMap tools for which additional problems, interventions, and intermediate goals and outcomes must be added; and can enhance creation of a completely individualized tool for complex, case-managed patients through immediate integration of developed standards of care.
- *It facilitates integration of pathways with physician order sets to allow the physician to verify the order set within the body of the CareMap tool on a daily/weekly/visit basis, making changes as necessary based on patient condition.* This would then be linked to and generate the medication administration record (MAR). This is a time-saving intervention for a number of personnel and could reduce dosage and transcription errors.
- *It provides concurrent data management for individual patients.* For example, it enables analysis of patient acuity, resources predicted versus resources consumed, current versus expected cost of care delivered within each account (for example, time spent in ICU, specialty, or general care unit) and dollars left to spend, clinical variances that have occurred and how they are being managed, and intermediate goals realized and outcomes achieved. This allows staff to monitor the balance of the patient's checkbook, to determine patient acuity/work load, to determine actions to be taken by all members of the health care team to meet the outcomes identified, and to provide a database for continuous quality

improvement processes. It also will enhance the clinician's ability to deliver high-quality care in a resource-constrained environment.

- *It provides a system for concurrent collection of variances.* It does this by forcing the clinician to choose a reason or cause and to create an action plan to address the variance before exiting the CareMap tool on the computer (demand field). The information can then be collated into an established report format generated at the end of each month with distribution to the appropriate individuals and committees for review. Relational database software programs must be designed to accommodate the goals to be accomplished with variance analysis. It is imperative that clinicians, managers, and administrators be able to investigate relational data within and across case types by such dimensions as age, sex, comorbidities, specific clinical problems, or issues such as pain management. Additionally, the clinical, qualitative data must be linked to fiscal data to determine the impact on cost.
- *It provides a structure for conducting action research by capturing preidentified or marked data elements on the CareMap tool as the patient is cared for.* It allows for testing clinical interventions as correlated with intermediate goals and outcomes. In this fashion, clinicians can measure scientifically the impact on quality and care outcomes of changes made to the care delivered.

Once the CareMap tool is computerized, clinicians can access databases to make efficient and effective decisions about patient care; reduce the repetitive, time-consuming activities of hand-tallying acuity measures; determine resource utilization and perform appropriateness review; determine concurrent cost outliers whose care must be managed; collate variance data and generate reports; and so on. As a result, time will be saved in reduced rework within and between disciplines in actions taken and information documented, errors in order transcription will be decreased, collaborative team efforts to achieve patient outcomes will be enhanced, and care will be more closely managed and cost and quality outliers monitored.

Three Examples of Successful CareMap Automation

Three institutions and one vendor have successfully integrated portions of the CareMap system with information technology. These are Vanderbilt University Medical Center, Nashville, Tennessee; the Hemet Valley Medical Center, Hemet, California; Baptist Health System, Birmingham, Alabama; and Hospital Computer System, Inc., Farmingdale, New Jersey, which is a vendor development initiative.

Vanderbilt University Medical Center

Pilon and Hill[5] describe Vanderbilt University Medical Center's personal computer (PC) stand-alone information system to integrate its collaborative path with a charting by exception system. The system starts with entry of admission data by the receptionist on the unit. The nurse then selects a collaborative path from the hard drive. Day one of the tool is customized for the patient through a hard-copy generation of the path and a flow sheet for data documentation. A charting by exception format is used. If the patient does not meet predicted activities identified on the collaborative path or assessment standards for the case type, a narrative note is written. The nurse must evaluate patient progress against clinical outcomes within each 24-hour time frame. If the outcomes are not being met, the variance system is initiated through a demand field. The variance reports are generated periodically for quality monitoring and improvement.

Hemet Valley Medical Center

The Hemet Valley Medical Center reported development of a mainframe system to support the use of coordinated patient outcome system across the continuum (from hospital to home care) and their integration into the order-entry and documentation systems.[6] According to John Hall and Derrick Spellman,[7,8] due to the interface between the multidisciplinary action plan (MAP) and order-entry systems, potential variances from expected tasks/activities or outcomes (as outlined on the MAP) and daily orders are automatically highlighted on the computer screen for the practitioner to affirm as a variance. Again, variance capture is assured. Variance is then tied to the quality management program.

Baptist Health System

Baptist Health System has undertaken a six-phase project to internally develop an automated CareMap. The product satisfies the following six key requirements:[9]

1. It integrates with other institutional patient care computer systems.
2. It adheres to strict, consistent relationships for presentation and analysis requirements.
3. It functions within current computer network and hardware.
4. It is the focal point for all clinical documentation.
5. It resides in an industry standard relational database.
6. It is stored on-line so quality improvement analysis can be conducted at any time.

Nurses, case managers, and, in the near future, ancillary clinicians document against the automated CareMap. Collated variance data are generated in a report format for the cardiovascular case managers to analyze. Variance charting against the CareMap is seen as only the beginning. The ultimate goal projected for the system is to tie all documentation back to the CareMap. The CareMap will then be updated automatically as vital signs, assessments, and results are entered. In the future cost will also be tied to each of the activities on the CareMap. The institutions may even predict staffing requirements from outlined interventions and outcomes to be achieved on a daily basis.

Hospital Computer System

Hospital Computer System, Inc. (HCS), has created INTERACTANT™ CareMap software. This technical application enables performance of a number of functions. For example:

- It supports the daily use of collaborative paths in clinical practice by allowing the clinician to view three periods at a time.
- It allows individualization of the CareMap tool to meet patient needs and insertion of detours.
- It supports multidisciplinary documentation and automates identification of caregiver and department.
- It provides necessary interface with HCS-driven registration, order-entry, and financial systems.
- It incorporates exception documentation.
- It contains a variance database capturing all outcomes and select interventions.
- It provides reports on aggregate and concurrent variance data.

This product greatly assists clinicians in evaluating quality and cost outcomes realized for both the individual patient and the aggregate patient population. A valuable software application, it demonstrates only a fraction of the integration that will be possible in the near future.

Review of the Institution's CareMap Educational Programs

Following development of the CareMap tool, the CareMap team often embarks on a review of the educational programs offered to patients. Typically, several issues become apparent, the most striking of which is that the educational sessions offered by different disciplines and the instructional materials they use vary widely in content and language. Because hospitalized patients retain only about 35 percent of information received, the team begins to question what information patients should receive and at what stages during their episode of illness. The team then determines the priority of issues to be discussed, the content to be taught, the consistent set of words to be used, and the disciplines responsible for various pieces of the program. Key components of this educational curriculum are then built into the teaching and outcome sections of the CareMap tool.

In designing CareMap tools, the team is challenged to evaluate the ability of staff to teach and of patients to learn the information presented within a specific time frame. For example, as postvaginal delivery length of stay has decreased to 24 hours, nurses have attempted to teach in 24 hours the same information taught traditionally in the acute care setting in a 72-hour time frame. In this case, the team might discuss the need to look at the entire pregnancy and to consider what information should be taught and at what stage along this continuum. The team might then completely redesign the educational curriculum to focus on the priority issues to be learned on infant and maternal care, as well as strengthen the consistency of educational content across geographical settings.

As a result, a very strong, consistent, and structured educational program that greatly benefits patients and families, conserves resources, and ensures achievement of outcomes is created. Additionally, when the tool is shared and reviewed with patients/families, it appears to enhance their satisfaction with the care delivered. As hospitals strive to gain market share and informed consumers raise their expectations, the need to collect performance data in expanded arenas becomes more obvious. In an era when patients are recovering postprocedure in the community rather than in the acute care setting, in addition to requesting information about the care they are to receive, patients/families are demanding input into the plan of care, adequate pain control, and better discharge planning.

To respond to these demands, several institutions are involving patients in focus groups designed for CareMap tool review. Patients are asked to discuss their needs, how best to meet their needs, and how to build their needs into the body of the CareMap tool. Involving patients enhances the hospital's ability to better meet their physical and emotional needs.

A number of institutions across the country have discovered the need to create patient-focused CareMap tools. Among these institutions are ScrippsHealth in San Diego, California; Presbyterian Hospital in Charlotte, North Carolina; United Samaritans Hospital in Danville, Illinois; and Shriner's Hospital for Crippled Children in Greenville, South Carolina. The tools are written in simplified language and include the key elements that patients must understand and participate in. The tools highlight what patients can expect from the health care team during hospitalization and what the health care team should expect from them. The tools are distributed in the physician's office, the preadmission testing area, or on admission to the hospital.

Conclusion

The strength of the CareMap system lies in its emphasis on evaluation of cost and quality outcomes. Integration of CareMap tools with the hospital's documentation system, information technology, and patient education will produce a number of benefits. These include decreased fragmentation in care; increased access to services; the ability to capture clinical and cost outcome data; the ability to better manage clinical and cost outliers; the ability to compare benchmark data on local, regional, and national levels; and the ability to conduct applied outcome research.

Although CareMap systems remain in development and constant evolution, it is clear that they are crucial to strengthening the patient–family–health care provider partnership. Thus, to ensure the promotion and maintenance of society's health, it is essential that ongoing commitment be made to outcome-based practice, cost containment, and the integration and automation of these systems.

References

1. Joint Commission on Accreditation of Hospitals. *Standards for Accreditation of Hospitals.* Oakbrook Terrace, IL: JCAHO, 1969.

2. Pozgar, G. D. *Legal Aspects of Healthcare Administration.* 4th Ed. Rockville, MD: Aspen Publishing, 1990.

3. Nolin, C. E., and Lang, C. G. *An Analysis of the Use and Effect of CareMap Tools in Medical Malpractice Litigation.* South Natick, MA: The Center for Case Management, Inc., 1994.

4. Zander, K. Dear vendor. *Computers in Healthcare* 14(6):34, June 1993.

5. Pilon, B. A., and Hill, M. Integration of Managed Care with Informational Systems. In: M. E. Mills, editor. *Information Management: Strategies and Support for Data Driven Decisions in Nursing and Health Care.* Springhouse, PA: Springhouse Corporation, 1995.

6. Hemet Valley Medical Center. *Managed Care Through Coordinated Care: Coordinated Patient Outcome System.* Palm Springs, CA: HVMC, 1991.

7. Spellman, D. Presentation at the *Expert User's Forum,* The Center for Case Management, at Charleston, South Carolina, Jan. 1992.

8. Hall, J. Personal conversation with Maria Hill, Dec. 16, 1994.

9. Rides, B., and Favor, G. Baptist Health System, Birmingham, AL. Letter. Dec. 16, 1994.

CHAPTER EIGHT

Case Management Designed for the Care Continuum

Kathleen Bower, DNSc

The effective management of patient care is assuming greater urgency in today's changing health care environment. Changes in reimbursement methodologies are contributing to the urgency, making continuum-based approaches to care a mandate for provider survival. The mandate is to view health care as a seamless system for patients at both the individual and aggregate levels. There is increasing recognition that fragmented care is ineffective in terms of quality and, ultimately, cost.

This chapter explores case management as a strategy for coordinating care across the care continuum. It describes the different case management models, the design of a case management system, and the role of the case manager within the system.

The Nature of the Care Continuum

The concept of continuum spans many dimensions, principally health/illness, time span, and locale. By its very nature, the continuum *is* the "big picture" created from many components. Focusing on the continuum generates a deeper understanding of the numerous and intricate interrelationships involved in providing patient care. Each provider of, and locale for, care is in a symbiotic relationship with all other providers and locales. Care provided at any earlier stage will almost always influence the current care process and, in turn, all subsequent care.

Originally, health care was provided on a continuum basis. The continuum focus was de facto, based on limited numbers of providers, treatment options, and sites for providing care. Recently, however, care has been fragmented by the increasing numbers and sophistication of treatment options and sites, which has resulted in an intricate, specialty-based system. Although recognizing the benefits of highly sophisticated specialties, the health care system is being deliberately transformed to tighten the coordination of patient care across disciplines, specialties, time, and locales. Thus, the health care system is recycling to once again acknowledge that managing the care continuum is critical to support quality and cost-effectiveness.

The shift is away from illness-based acute care and toward a focus on health, wellness, and the effective support of ill individuals at the lowest, most appropriate level of service intensity. In part, this is based on the belief that prevention and early intervention produce a higher level of quality at a lower cost.

Continuum-focused approaches to care seek the best timing and place for all the activities involved. As demonstrated in figure 8-1, acute care provides the opportunity for health restoration and little else. Longer-term issues such as recovery, health maintenance, and health promotion occur outside the acute care setting, generally in the community. By linking the components into an integrated continuum, patients are more likely to receive information and interventions when and where they are most receptive to them. This is especially urgent in the emerging health care environment because of the rapidly shrinking length of stay in acute care settings.

By strategizing the entire continuum, access to care can be more effectively established. Although everyone currently has access to care, that care may not be available until an acute or life-threatening (and usually costly) issue has emerged. Thus, access to lower-intensity, lower-cost care must be established throughout the continuum.

Strategies for Coordinating Care

The major approach to improve quality and cost-effectiveness is to coordinate patient care effectively. Case management is one of several, related strategies designed to accomplish this. Although in itself very powerful, the case management approach can be enhanced when used with other approaches or strategies such as resource management or critical paths/CareMap tools.

A well-integrated process for coordinating care includes multiple strategies, including those outlined in figure 8-2, and each strategy has a specific role within the health care organization. To achieve both effectiveness and efficiency, it is important to link strategies to the appropriate patient population and the appropriate circumstances. Figure 8-3 shows the relationships between some of these strategies, locales, and time spans.

Figure 8-1. Care over the Continuum

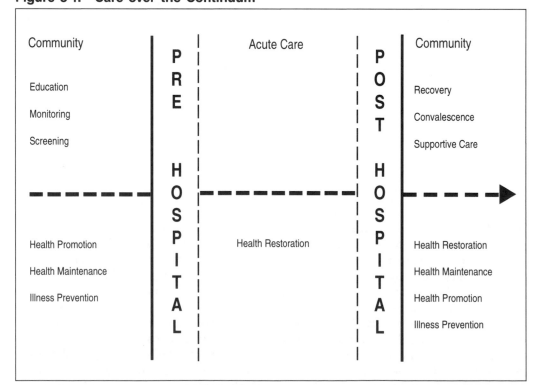

Reprinted, with permission, from Carondelet St. Mary's Hospital, Tucson, Arizona. Copyright C. Falk, Carondelet St. Mary's Hospital.

Figure 8-2. Dimensions of and Strategies for Care Coordination

Dimensions	Patients	Strategy
Resource Need based on: • Diverse sources for payment of health care • Efficient identification of and access to appropriate postdischarge resources	All	**Resource Management** The process of identifying, confirming, and negotiating benefits and resources for the patient. This includes screening for benefits eligibility; communicating with the patient and the health care team, especially when benefits and the plan are out of alignment; communicating and negotiating with the payers regarding the anticipated plan of care; identifying postdischarge needs and benefits and arranging for posthospitalization care and community resources.
Program Involves patient populations with sufficient volume that have similar, recurring, patternable needs for services across their episode of care.	Percent varies by nature of the organization.	**Program Management** The process of developing a formal system of care, including services and resources, for an identified population of patients with similar needs. Within program management, consistent availability of services is developed and a means of patient access to the program is established.
Unit/Area/Discipline Based Need based on the reduced length of stay, emphasis on efficient use of resources, and minimizing fragmentation within a given geographic area of care (such as nursing unit or home health).	All	**Care Coordination (Care Management)** The process and system developed to organize and orchestrate the care of all patients within a specific geographic area in such a way that it is directed toward meeting desired/anticipated unit-based outcomes within an appropriate length of stay and resource utilization. In nursing, it is the nursing care delivery system that is established.
Episode Based Some patients require more concentrated coordination of care throughout some or all of their episode of care, spanning geographic care areas and bridging the various services and disciplines involved. **Continuum Based** A small percentage of patients require support coordinating and managing care needs for long periods of time. Individuals typically have chronic health issues that are often accompanied by complicating factors such as social or economic issues.	Less than 20%	**Case Management** A clinical system that focuses on the accountability of an individual or group for coordinating a patient's care (or group of patients) across an episode or continuum of care, ensuring and facilitating the achievement of quality, clinical and in financial outcomes, negotiating, procuring, and coordinating services and resources needed by the patient/family; intervening at key points (and/or at significant variances from the plan of care) for individual patients; addressing and resolving consistent issues that have a negative quality–cost impact; and creating opportunities and systems to enhance outcomes.
Coordination of Plan via a standardized plan	60–80%	**Critical Path/CareMap Tool** A cause-and-effect grid which identifies expected patient/family and staff behaviors against a time line for a case type or otherwise defined homogeneous population. A critical path/CareMap tool reflects the best-practice patterns of the clinicians of all key disciplines and departments across the episode that author the content. They are used to coordinate, plan, deliver, monitor, document, and review care concurrently. Variances from the tool are identified, addressed, and resolved at the individual and aggregate levels. Aggregate variance data are used retrospectively for Continuous Quality Improvement.

Figure 8-3. Expanding Scope of Accountability

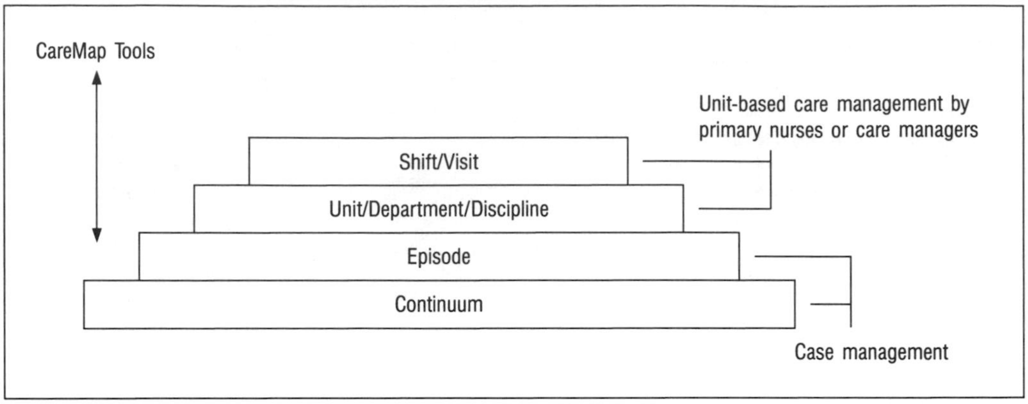

The Case Management Strategy

As previously noted, case management is one of the strategies for coordinating the care of patients with complex issues over an episode or continuum. Following is a working definition of this strategy:

> A clinical system that focuses on the accountability of an identified individual or group for coordinating a patient's care (or group of patients) across an episode or continuum; negotiating, procuring, and coordinating services and resources needed by the patient/family; ensuring and facilitating the achievement of quality, clinical, and cost outcomes; intervening at key points for individual patients; addressing and resolving patterns of issues that have a negative quality–cost impact; and creating opportunities and systems to enhance outcomes.

The goal of case management is to achieve desired clinical and cost outcomes by providing a well-coordinated experience for patients/families and by synchronizing care activities of multiple disciplines and providers.

Case Management Models

Many models for case management have emerged. As figure 8-4 shows, they can differ according to a number of criteria, including:

- Payment source
- Location
- Discipline and/or model
- Time frame

Although each model is listed separately, they can be combined to establish a case management system. For example, a community-based nurse case management system combines case management by location and case management by discipline. A useful case management system for an organization incorporates several models or approaches. The most important consideration is to establish a system that addresses the needs and characteristics of multiple patient populations as well as the organization.

Despite the multiple approaches to case management, five key features emerge. These are that case management is a system that:

1. Focuses on patients/families with complex issues
2. Revolves around negotiating, coordinating, and procuring services needed by the focus patients/families
3. Is based on building relationships and developing networks
4. Involves the use of a clinical reasoning process
5. Is episode and/or continuum focused

Case Management Patients

Case management is a resource in that it requires an investment of staff, time, benefits, equipment, and supplies. As a resource, case management is focused on patient populations who will benefit most from the service. Most often, these are individuals who

Figure 8-4. Case Management Models

By Payment Source

Internal Case Management that is sponsored by care providers (such as hospitals, Home Health, Rehabilitation facilities). This outline of Case Management models will focus on internal or provider-based systems.

External: Case Management that is sponsored by third-party payers such as commercial insurers or HMOs.

By Location

Community Based: Designed to address multidimensional needs and issues of individuals who are the community. This model of Case Management may be sponsored by a hospital or by other organizations within the community (such as Home Health or Visiting Nurse).

Hospital Based: Case Management that begins with admission to the hospital or other care facility (or with identification of the need for admission) and continues until the patient is discharged from the hospital, working with the patient and staff within each area in which the patient receives care. This model of Case Management may also incorporate postdischarge follow-up such as telephone calls, home visits, and/or meeting the patient during a posthospital physician or ambulatory visit.

Unit Based: Case Management is *not* unit based and so this designation is a misnomer. This approach to managing care is more accurately known as Care Coordination and focuses on effectively managing patient care during the time that a patient is located on/in a given geographical area (such as a hospital unit or within home health). Alternative job titles: Patient Care Coordinator, Care Manager.

By Discipline and/or Model

Utilization Management/Quality Management/Discharge Planning: Focuses on efficient management of resources and on effective movement of patients toward discharge. Alternative job title: Patient Resource Coordinator.

Clinical: Case Management that focuses on the need for coordinating the resources and services needed by *patients* presenting with complex problems resulting from an interaction of physical, emotional, psychological, spiritual, social, and/or economic issues.

Social: Designed to meet the needs of individuals with complex or complicated social or psychosocioeconomic issues. Most often provided by

Social Workers. This model of Case Management may also be sponsored by community organizations such as senior citizen groups.

Nurse Case Management: Case Management that is provided by registered nurses, generally under the sponsorship and management of a department of nursing within a hospital or other health care organization.

By Time Frame

Episode Based: Case Management that begins with the identification of the need for enhanced coordination (example, during a prehospital screening process) of services and resources for individuals, and continues until the individual no longer requires care for that health issue. Episode based indicates that the Case Management process is *time limited.*

Continuum Based: Case Management that begins with the identification of the need for enhanced coordination of services and resources for individuals and continues *infinitely* until the issues are resolved or until death.

Reprinted, with permission, from The Center for Case Management, South Natick, MA.

present with complex issues rather than acute health care situations. In this case, *complexity* is the interaction of diverse elements such as health, social, emotional, economical, and/or spiritual issues.

Patients within priority populations usually include those who:

- Incur high costs
- Present with significant socioeconomic, psychological, emotional, and/or spiritual issues
- Are at high risk for encountering major disruptions in their plan of care
- Experience multiple hospital or emergency department admissions or require numerous visits to the offices of physicians or other providers
- Receive care from several disciplines and/or multiple physicians

Often patients selected for case management are those for whom critical paths are difficult to create because their care is not patternable or predictable. Case-managed patients have an intense need to have their care coordinated, especially across an episode or continuum spanning care sites and providers. A reasonable estimate of the number of patients within a given facility who will need case management services is less than 20 percent.

The Role of Case Manager

The case manager role is multidimensional in which clinical skills synergistically interact with management and interpersonal skills. Figure 8-5 provides a sample, generic role description that demonstrates the range of activities encompassed within this position.

Within the context of complex patient situations, the providers who most often take on the case manager role are from the disciplines of nursing or social work. Providers from other disciplines, such as psychology or physical therapy, may assume the case manager role depending on the needs of the patient population.

The complexity of patient and system issues and the skills related to their management increasingly supports an advanced level of educational preparation for the case manager role. Although individuals with varying levels of educational preparation currently function as case managers, based on the degree of complexity of services, the minimum preparation needs to be at the baccalaureate level and ideally at the master's level.

In addition to educational preparation, case managers must accrue a body of knowledge and skills to function effectively in the role. A sample of the skills and knowledge related to case management is provided in figure 8-6. Because new case managers may not demonstrate all the desired skills and knowledge upon assuming the role, a structured, organized plan for ongoing assessment and addressing learning needs must be in place.

As a structural issue, case managers need flexibility in terms of time and location to manage the varying and intense needs of patients across the multiple sites in which they receive care. The flexibility required of this position most often calls for an individual whose focus is exclusively on case management activities and who will not be distracted by the demands of additional roles. Whether a case manager can effectively function on a part-time schedule depends on the needs and characteristics of the patients and the match between the proposed schedule and patient needs.

Caseload size varies among settings. Three factors influence caseload size:

1. The complexity of the patient population
2. The amount of direct care provided by the case manager
3. The number and size of geographical areas involved

Figure 8-5. Case Manager Role Functions

General Role Description

Coordinates, negotiates, procures, and manages the care of complex patients to facilitate achievement of quality and cost patient outcomes. Works collaboratively with interdisciplinary staff internal and external to the organization. Participates in quality improvement and evaluation processes related to the management of patient care.

Role Functions

1. Within the organization's established criteria for Case Management services, identifies appropriate patients for Case Management for the service of area covered.
2. Develops a network of the usual services and disciplines required by the typical patient within the caseload.
3. Establishes a system for coordinating the caseload patient's care throughout the entire continuum of care, spanning each geographic area in which care is provided.
4. Establishes methods for tracking patients' progress through the health care systems within the entire episode or continuum of care.
5. Maintains a working knowledge of the requirements of the payers most frequently seen with the patient population.
6. Maintains a working knowledge of the resources available in the community for patient/family needs.
7. Demonstrates flexibility and creativity in identifying resources to meet patient/family needs.
8. Establishes a means of communicating and collaborating with physicians, other team members, the patient payers, and administrators.
9. Explores strategies to reduce length of stay and resource consumption within the case-managed patient populations, implements them and documents the results.
10. Evaluates the effects of case management on the targeted patient populations.
11. Introduces self to the patient/family, explains the Case Manager role, and provides them with a business card.
12. Assesses the patients within the caseload to identify needs, issues, resources, and care goals.
13. In conjunction with the patient/family, other members of the health care team, the payer, and available resource:

    a. Formulates a plan to address assessed needs and issues.
    b. Implements the plan.
    c. Evaluates the effectiveness of the plan in meeting the established care goals.
    d. Revises the plan as needed to reflect changing needs, issues, and goals.

14. Manages each patient's transitions through the system and transfers accountability to the appropriate person or agency upon discharge from the Case Management service.
15. Maintains appropriate documentation of patient care and progress within the established plan.
16. Coordinates, negotiates, and procures services and disciplines needed by patients/families.
17. Communicates with other members of the health team regarding the patient's needs, plan, and response to care.
18. Works collaboratively with staff members from the disciplines and areas (such as nursing units) involved in the patients' care.
19. Identifies the need for, arranges for, and conducts health care team meetings when necessary to facilitate the coordination of complex services and resources.
20. Educates health team colleagues about Case Management, including the role and the unique needs of the case-managed patient populations.
21. As a member of the Case Management Practice:

    a. Seeks and provides peer consultation about cases that are presenting problems and/or experiencing significant deviations from the plan of care.
    b. Consistently attends meetings of the practice group and participates in them.
    c. Participates in regular peer review regarding the management of the caseload.
    d. Participates in Quality Improvement and evaluation processes related to the Case Management Practice.
    e. Arranges for and participates in coverage during long, short, and unexpected absences of self and other Case Managers.

22. Reviews pertinent literature about case types managed and shares with peers and colleagues as needed.

Reprinted, with permission, from The Center for Case Management, South Natick, MA.

Figure 8-6.   Minimal Knowledge and Skill Components of the Case Manager's Role

---

Knowledge

- Health care finance and economics
- General knowledge of the health care system
- Requirements of the most frequently encountered payers
- Available patient care resources within and external to the organization

Skills

Clinical

- Clinical reasoning process
- Specialized knowledge required by the specific patient population

Interpersonal

- Communication (verbal and written)
- Collaboration
- Participation as a team member

Management

- Negotiation
- Project management
- Quality improvement
- Priority setting
- Time management
- Outcomes management
- Consultation
- Conflict management
- Managing meetings
- Data analysis and management

Assuming moderate complexity, minimal direct interventions by the case manager, and reasonable geography, caseload size typically ranges between 20 and 35 active patients. There may be many additional patients on inactive status who do not currently need case management services but who have potential needs if their condition changes.

The Case Manager–Patient Relationship

The pivotal element in case management is the process of establishing effective relationships with patients/families, associated providers of care, and payers. The case manager–patient relationship begins when a patient is identified as needing case management services and a referral is initiated. At that point, the case manager screens the patient by reviewing the case to date and, in many cases, by interacting with the patient/family. This leads to a decision about whether the patient will benefit from case management services or whether other sources of support would be more appropriate. Usually, patient agreement for case management services is implicitly or explicitly obtained as well.

Once the patient is admitted to the service, the case manager completes a more thorough assessment building on earlier assessments of the patient's situation by the various members of the health care team and, often, by the payer. The assessment includes an identification of goals, resources, and limitations. Goals are negotiated based on the assessment with input from the patient, related providers, and the payer. A plan for reaching the goals is established, including a time line. If a critical path is in use, the case manager reviews it with direct care staff and provides input.

The Case Manager and the Case Management Process

The case manager orchestrates implementation of the plan using a number of approaches. He or she may negotiate directly with the service providers or may arrange with others (such as direct care providers) to do so. In some situations, the case manager may actually provide some of the interventions. However, this approach is increasingly rare because it may interfere with the case manager's availability to coordinate the care of multiple patients.

Establishing and maintaining a network within which needed activities and services can be provided with maximum efficiency is a key case manager function in the implementation stage. Networks are developed to respond to the needs of individual patients. A sample network is provided in figure 8-7. When a case manager's practice has a consistent focus (for example, oncology or maternity), core members of the network are identified for the population and additional members added to respond to the specific needs of individual patients.

As care progresses, the case manager closely monitors the time lines and effectiveness of planned interventions in relation to the established goals. This is accomplished by assessing and interacting with the patient/family and communicating with the network members. It also may include arranging for and leading a meeting of the health care team to discuss and resolve emerging issues.

Revisions to the plan are made promptly when planned activities do not lead to desired outcomes or when the patient's situation or condition changes. The case manager again negotiates revisions to the plan and/or goals with the patient/family, network members, and the payer.

The case management process and case manager–patient relationship continue until either the goals are met or the patient's situation no longer requires case management services. This time line may extend over weeks, months, or even years. When the case manager's services are no longer needed by the patient, the patient is discharged from the caseload. Sometimes the patient is placed on inactive status until needs reemerge. Patients also may be transferred to another support system—for example, when a patient moves from the community served by the case manager. Each phase of the case management process is documented in the patient record, using the system established by the organization.

The Case Management System

At the individual patient level, case management is both a role and a process. At the organizational level, it is a system. As a system, case management must be developed

Figure 8-7. Sample Case Management Network

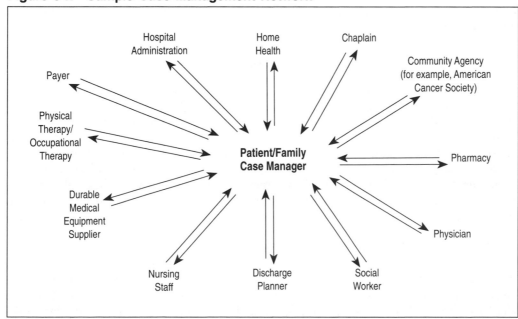

and managed. Development includes responding to immediate patient and organizational concerns. It also includes a view of case management as an evolving system that must be adjusted periodically to better fit changing needs and issues.

Designing the System

The process of initiating and revising a case management system begins with identifying priority patients and patient populations. Subsequent system development revolves around four factors:

1. The needs and characteristics of the focus populations
2. The needs and characteristics of the organization
3. Actual and potential resources within the organization
4. The goals of case management at the organizational and specific patient population levels

These factors guide many decisions regarding the case management system.

Two issues that must be addressed are how long and where the case manager will interact with the patients. For example, the case manager may be involved with the patient primarily during hospitalization, with minimal or no contact before or after hospital care. Alternatively, case management interventions may begin long before (or even be unrelated to) an acute care stay and continue for a defined period of time thereafter. Chronically ill patients may need to receive most of their case management services in the community over the course of years.

As the shape of the case management service emerges, the question of how to organize the system becomes important. A related issue is that of setting up the reporting relationship. A variety of options exist in this area. These include:

- Establishing a separate case management department
- Decentralizing the reporting of case managers to product line administrators
- Setting up reporting relationships within clinical or financial divisions

The most important consideration is that, to be successful, case management must address the agendas of multiple and diverse audiences. One way to accomplish this may be to establish a matrix structure with clear delineation of accountability and communication expectations.

Assigning Patients to the System

When a system involving two or more case managers is established, decisions are needed as to how the patients will be assigned. One approach is to assign patients to case managers in a rotating fashion as vacancies occur in caseloads. In many situations, it may be advantageous to focus individual case managers' practices along specific patient populations. The populations may be defined through characteristics such as diagnosis, body system, geography (especially in community-based case management), physician, or age. This approach facilitates development of a deeper knowledge base by the case manager and establishment of more consistent, and ultimately more effective, relationships with other providers involved in the patient population's care. In any assignment methodology, flexibility is crucial to maintaining continuity of service to case-managed patients.

Likewise, in any system with more than one case manager, it may be useful to develop case management as a group practice, regardless of the reporting relationships of individual case managers. A *group practice* is a formal or informal structure that brings together all the case managers within the organization on a regular basis. The goals of this structure are to:

- Ensure consistent information sharing between case managers and between organizational administrators and managers
- Develop consistency of role definition and system processes among case managers dealing with diverse patient populations
- Provide a forum for structured and unstructured education and development of the case managers individually and as a group

In a group practice, case managers can establish and solidify a number of issues. These include:

- Consistent procedures, processes, standards, and protocols for the case management process within the organization
- A system for peer consultation and review
- Approaches to evaluating the outcomes of case management
- Educational needs and ways to meet them
- Communication networks within and external to practice members
- A system for cross coverage during planned and unanticipated case manager absences
- A consistent quality measurement and improvement process for case management within the organization

However, it is important to remember that the ongoing usefulness of the case management system depends on how well it is managed. This involves attending to the elements of effective system design as outlined in figure 8-8. Briefly, these elements include:

- A clear definition of case management for the organization
- An outline of specific case management goals
- Evidence of the organization's support for the case management system
- A clear definition of the case manager role
- A well-defined outline of the case management process
- A method for addressing the developmental needs of case managers
- An established process for quality measurement and improvement
- An established process for evaluating the case management process and outcomes

The system's usefulness also relies on a vision of case management as an evolving process that must be regularly reshaped to meet changing patient and organizational needs.

Conclusion

Case management is a powerful approach to managing the care of complex patient populations over their care continuum. The need for case management will grow in the health care environment of the future. As health care reform continues to evolve, new case management models also will emerge that respond to the changing issues.

Case management is a valuable resource within an organization. As such, it must be developed and nurtured in a planned way. This requires careful management of the system and ongoing development of the individuals who assume the case manager role. An effective system will not emerge through serendipity. It is a sufficiently productive process to warrant an investment of time and resources in careful development.

Figure 8-8. Anatomy of an Effective Case Management Design

Case Management is defined clearly for the organization.

Goals are specifically outlined for the organization.

Case Management is concretely supported by the organization as evidenced by:

- The inclusion of Case Management in the organization's strategic plan and/or mission statement.
- A functioning, administrative level Steering Committee.
- Resources appropriately allocated to the Case Management process.

The Case Manager's role is defined.

- Integration with other roles is clarified.

The Case Management process is outlined, including the referral and discharge process and criteria.

- Supporting documentation and referrals have been developed.

The developmental needs of Case Managers are addressed in an organized way:

- Knowledge and skill needs are assessed regularly.
- An orientation process is outlined and provided to each new Case Manager.
- Ongoing developmental needs are addressed through such mechanisms as:
  —A structured performance appraisal process.
  —A mechanism for peer review.
  —A formal, regularly scheduled format for case presentation and supervision.

A process for Quality Measurement and Improvement is in place.

A process for evaluating the process and outcomes associated with Case Management is established.

- Data are available and in a useful format.
- Evaluation criteria at both the process and outcome levels have been established.
  —Outcomes related to both quality and cost are assessed.
  —Significant trends are addressed on a regular basis.

Reprinted, with permission, from The Center for Case Management, South Natick, MA.

CHAPTER NINE

Program Evaluation

Mary Crabtree Tonges and Judith L. Brett, PhD

Care management and case management are powerful tools for improving the quality and controlling the cost of patient care through increased coordination and continuity of care delivery; however, successful implementation of these initiatives usually necessitates considerable organizational change requiring the investment of time, effort, and other valuable resources. Thus, it is critical that a process be developed to evaluate program outcomes so that organizations implementing these initiatives can ensure that their goals are being met and their investment is justified. When initiating an evaluation effort, two key questions must be addressed: (1) What do evaluators expect to achieve? and (2) How will they know that they have achieved it?

This chapter provides guidance in developing an evaluation plan for care/case management programs. It discusses development of a conceptual framework or model, the role of program objectives, and the activities to be included in plan development. It also describes how to work with qualitative and quantitative data, and offers recommendations on how to make care/case management evaluation work most effectively.

Conceptual Frameworks

Conceptual frameworks identify and organize key elements within an area of interest and can thus guide the development of programs and their objectives. Although not always explicitly stated, ideas about important elements and expected relationships underlie every effort to design a new patient care delivery system. Displaying the expected interrelationships among variables within a conceptual framework schematically helps guide decisions about what to measure.

One approach to conceptualizing case management is shown in figure 9-1. This model suggests that evaluation of care/case management programs can be structured around the examination of outcomes for patients, caregivers, and institutions. The model is supported by a review of the objectives for care/case management programs identified in the literature, which indicates that they consistently center on improved patient, caregiver, and institutional outcomes.[1-3]

Organizational interventions such as restructuring systems of care in hospitals frequently are critiqued as being atheoretical.[4] In other words, they appear to have been developed out of thin air, without reference to a well-supported framework that would explain why they were designed in a particular way. Thus, it is important to make the mental model guiding development of the care management program explicit by articulating a conceptual framework.

Program Objectives

A very important part of care/case management program development is to set objectives, that is, to formally identify the program's purpose and goals. When the evaluation process is initiated, these original objectives must be revisited. Although every organization is unique in some ways and may have certain institution-specific goals, the objectives set for care/case management programs generally share a common theme. Following is a list of objectives that are common to most care/case management programs:

- To decrease cost and length of stay (LOS) per case type
- To improve patient outcomes
- To increase the consistency of patient care processes
- To increase patient/family satisfaction
- To increase professional staff satisfaction

Determining the extent to which these goals have been attained is often the central focus of evaluation.

Figure 9-1.   Case Management as a Bottom-Line Management and Quality of Care Delivery Model: Features of the Process and Their Relationship with Model Outcomes

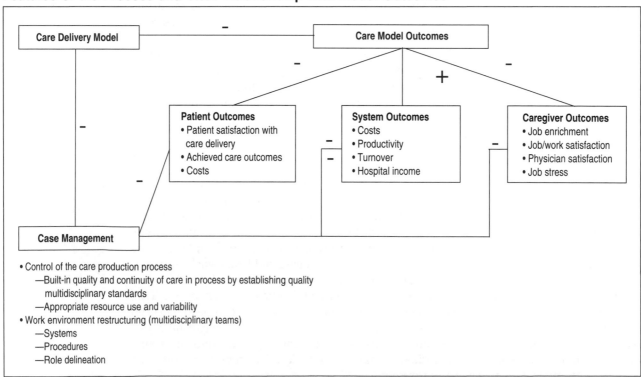

Note: The horizontal lines depict the relationships between process and outcomes; the signs on the lines relate to the direction of the relationship (positive or negative). The vertical lines depict select indication for the abstract constructs of care delivery model and care model outcomes.

Reprinted, with permission, from Olivas, G. S., and others. Case management: a bottom-line care delivery model, part 1: the concept. *Journal of Nursing Administration*, 19(11):19, 1989.

Program Evaluation as a Research Design

A *research design* is "a plan for conducting a study in such a way as to answer certain questions."[5] Designs differ in the amount of control that is exercised and provide the basis for different types of inferences. (For example, findings from a correlational study can suggest that there is a relationship between two variables, x and y, in which they increase together; however, a more controlled design would be needed to determine that x causes y to increase.) Thus, different designs are used for different purposes.

Major Types of Designs

Examples of the major types of designs provide a context for discussing program evaluation and understanding what it is and is not. Following are the most common types of design:

- *Nonexperimental design:* This type of design (for example, a case study of the implementation of CareMaps) provides a description of effects. Because variables are not controlled, this type of design is weak in providing evidence regarding the cause or impact of an intervention.
- *Relational research:* This type of design examines relationships between variables and analyzes how they vary together, but does not test the causality involved in the relationship (for example, correlation between the implementation of case management and nurses' job satisfaction).
- *Quasi-experimental design:* This type of design is more controlled but lacks some of the characteristics of pure experimental design (for example, it may use naturally occurring groups such as staff on a patient care unit rather than randomly assign subjects to experimental or control groups).
- *Experiments:* This type of design employs tightly controlled conditions and is used to test cause-and-effect relationships (for example, patients from the same case type are randomly assigned to case management or a control group).

The various types of design can be thought of as positioned on a continuum, beginning with nonexperimental designs at one end, moving through survey and correlational research and quasi-experimental designs, and ending with the experimental approach. Moving along the continuum from nonexperimental to experimental, the amount of control exerted by the researcher increases. Program evaluation is near the lower-control end of this range. It provides assessment and description of the degree to which a program achieves intended objectives but does not explain the causes of the results.

Program evaluation considers interventions from a larger perspective that "acknowledges potentially diffuse and multiple consequences."[6] This approach has been defined as "a set of procedures designed to systematically collect valid descriptive and judgmental information with regard to the ways in which a planned change effort has altered (or failed to alter) organizational processes."[7]

Key Features of Program Evaluation

Three of the key features of the program evaluation perspective are:[8]

1. A systemswide view
2. Measurements throughout the process
3. The acknowledged role of subjectivity

Thus, program evaluation generally entails the collection of data that represent the perspectives of multiple stakeholders, provides continuing measurement to assess whether the program is being implemented as intended and to identify changes in the effects over time, and "balances rigor and pragmatism" in that evaluators and managers agree on a plan that is rigorous enough to allow for some firm conclusions but is not so complex that it disrupts operations.[9]

The program evaluation approach is more concerned with results than the process through which inputs are converted into outcomes. This is why, as previously noted, the causes of outcomes are not explained. This aspect of program evaluation can be described by saying that the conversion process remains hidden within a "black box."

More sophisticated approaches to program evaluation are comparative. Instead of evaluating whether an intervention is better than no intervention, the relative merits of alternatives are considered. For example, it is fairly well established that having a case manager is more effective than not having a case manager, but who is the most effective case manager[10] and under what circumstances?

Principles and Processes of Evaluation Research

Polit and Hungler[11] describe *evaluation research* as an applied form of research that has as its goal the assessment or evaluation of the success of a program. According to Wood,[12] program evaluation does not fit into any one level of research but, rather, usually has characteristics of several levels. Of primary importance in choosing a research design is that it be based on the care/case management program's objectives.

Using an evaluation design instead of a more controlled research design does not necessarily mean choosing a less rigorous form of scientific testing. An experimental design often is inappropriate for real-life programs, or may be unethical in situations where a new program already exists and random assignment may exclude persons. However, to make interpretation of the effects of the program being studied as clear as possible, it is important to incorporate into an evaluation research design as many control techniques of experimental research as possible.

Wood[13] identifies four assumptions that are important to designs for program evaluation. These are:

1. Measurable objectives exist.
2. Methods or tools to measure the variables are available.
3. Objectives can be assigned priorities and be weighted according to their value to the project.
4. Sufficient control subjects exist to enable statistical testing to determine whether the program made a difference.

Operationalizing Objectives

The first and perhaps most critical part of all program evaluation is that of identifying, or operationalizing, the program objectives. Program objectives may be as general as "to improve quality" or as specific as "to decrease the turnover of registered nurses by 50 percent." Shigemitsu and Tsushima[14] listed six goals in their evaluation of nurse-managed care. These are:

1. To facilitate achievement of expected patient outcomes
2. To facilitate early discharge within an appropriate LOS
3. To promote appropriate and/or reduced utilization of resources
4. To promote collaborative practice, coordination, and continuity of care
5. To promote professional development and satisfaction of hospital-based registered nurses
6. To direct the contributions of all care providers toward achievement of patient outcomes

Whatever the intent of the program, to evaluate its achievements, the program evaluator must develop a clear understanding of its objectives.

Potential sources of objectives include program documents that may have been developed as part of the program approval process. For example, computer information system projects frequently are preceded by development of a request for proposal (RFP). This document includes the specifications for the system and identifies what it should do. Measurement of the system's performance against the initial specifications provides information about whether the system installed is what was proposed.

Vendor materials frequently make claims about the advantages of their systems or equipment. Often their claims (such as, "decreases costs," "saves nurses time," or "provides better quality of care") become incorporated in a project proposal as anticipated outcomes.

Another source of objectives are the administrators or leaders assigned responsibility for implementing the program. Usually these personnel have been involved in formulating and designing the program and thus should be able to articulate its objectives. Whether explicitly stated or inherent in the expected outcomes, the program's intended objectives must be ascertained prior to the start of the evaluation process.

Selecting Measurement Tools and Collecting Data

The second most critical step in program evaluation is that of establishing ways to measure goal achievement. Questionnaires and instruments are often used to accomplish this. Quantitative data such as costs or days spent in a hospital also are examples of measures. As in any research study, it is essential to the future acceptance of the program that the measurement tools or measures selected have evidence of reliability and validity.

Reliability refers to the accuracy and consistency of information obtained from a questionnaire. Reliability data about the instruments used should be included in the evaluation report. Questionnaires that do not provide reliable results (that is, results that can be duplicated if the conditions of the study were unchanged) should not be used. Techniques for improving reliability include ensuring that the questionnaire's instructions are clear and well understood and increasing the number of items. Test–retest and internal consistency reliability assessments are not difficult to complete and should be done each time an instrument is used. A rule of thumb in selecting instruments is that internal consistency should be at least .80. (Mishel[15] offers additional information on reliability assessment for instrument development and use.)

Validity is the degree to which a questionnaire measures what it is purported to measure. A patient satisfaction questionnaire is said to have validity if the result is directly related to the patient's "true" state of satisfaction. One way to ascertain test validity is to establish *content validity*. This is done by having a number of experts on the content of the questionnaire review it and agree that it measures the purpose intended. Another type of validity is *construct validity*. Construct validity is established by hypothesizing about the results of the questionnaire in a certain situation. For example, if a measure of job satisfaction is used in a situation of poor working conditions, high absenteeism, and high personnel turnover, it could be hypothesized that the satisfaction score will be low. If upon testing the score were found to be low, this would provide evidence of construct validity for the instrument as a measure of job satisfaction.

Examples of tools used in collaborative care program evaluation studies are listed in figure 9-2. Another good resource for tools and instruments, as well as for discussions on outcomes research issues, is the publication of the proceedings of the patient outcomes research conference sponsored by the National Center for Nursing Research.[16] Books of tools for different types of measurement purposes are also available in college libraries; a reference librarian can assist with locating this material.

Figure 9-2. Tools for Evaluating Program Outcomes

	Outcome	Applicable Tool	Reference
Essential	Patients' clinical outcomes	CareMap standards of care	
	Length of stay	CareMap and/or internal reports	
	Cost per case	Internal reports	
Desirable	Patient satisfaction	Koerner's Patient Satisfaction Survey	Koerner, B. L., Cohen, J. R., and Armstrong, D. N. Collaborative practice and patient satisfaction: impact and selected outcomes. *Evaluation and the Health Professions* 8:229–321, 1985.
	Patient satisfaction	Adaptation of Risser Patient Satisfaction Survey	Atwood, J., and Hinshaw, A. *Anticipated Turnover among Nursing Staff.* [DHHS Publication No. RO1 NU00908.] Tucson: University Medical Center Corporation, Nursing Department, 1984.
	Staff satisfaction	Index of Job Satisfaction	Brayfield, A., and Rothe, H. An index of job satisfaction. *Journal of Applied Psychology* 35:307–11, 1951.
	Nurse–physician collaboration	Collaborative Practice Scale	Weiss, S. J., and Davis, H. P. Validity and reliability of the Collaborative Practice Scales. *Nursing Research* 34:299–305, 1982.
	Job stress	Kinzel Stress Level Test	Kinzel, F. L. What's your stress level? *NurseLife* 2(2):54–55, 1982.
	Level of function	Role Functioning Scale	Green, R. S., and Gracely, E. J. Selecting a rating scale for evaluating services to the chronically medically ill. *Community Mental Health Journal* 23(2):91–102, 1987.
	Quality of life	Quality of Life Scale	Test, M. A., and Stein, L. I. Community treatment of the chronic patient: research overview. *Schizophrenia bulletin* 4(3):350–64, 1978.

Regardless of whether they are "homemade" or borrowed, the tools, instruments, and questionnaires selected should have an obvious relationship to the goals and objectives of the program being evaluated. For example, in the Shigemitsu and Tsushima study[17] referred to earlier, the data and measurement tools listed below were used to assess achievement of the study's goals. Some were developed specifically for the study and others had been used before. These measurement tools included:

- Patient satisfaction and outcome questionnaires
- LOS comparisons
- Patient charges
- Weiss Collaborative Practice Scale for nurses and physicians[18]
- Kinzel job stress scale,[19] self-ratings of competency, and personal and professional satisfaction scale
- Care management tools such as critical paths and variance reports

Although the authors did not report data about the validity and reliability of the questionnaires, it should be noted that the measures related directly to the stated goals and objectives of the study.

Finally, Isaac and Michael's caution concerning operationalizing objectives should be seriously considered in all program evaluation efforts. They wrote that:

Although great care should be taken to insure that the objectives are substantive and worthwhile, [and]...that the measures themselves are sound and valid, once the program design is complete, one fact acquires paramount significance. The measures on which the successful attainment will be based have now become the operational definition of the objectives.[20]

The questionnaires and statistics identified will be capable of measuring only what is built into them and nothing else. Any materials, substance, or value that is not built into these measures will not appear in the analysis. Thus, identifying measures for program evaluation is critical to analyzing program success or failure.

Other principles of good data collection and management should be followed. For example:

- *Data collection forms should be clear, concise, and easy to follow.* All data collection forms and processes should be piloted, preferably by the evaluator. This maximizes the likelihood that the required data will be collected in the most efficient manner.
- *An effort should be made to avoid inventing or developing a new measurement tool.* Whenever possible, an instrument should be used that has been developed for a research study, used several times, and evaluated for reliability and validity each time. Usually authors are willing to grant permission to use an instrument, particularly if the borrower is willing to share the results of his or her own validity and reliability testing.
- *It is important to be realistic about what can be accomplished during an evaluation process.* Some data are just too expensive to obtain, requiring too many man-hours to collect to be an affordable part of the evaluation.
- *It is equally important not to overestimate what is available from an information system.* Sometimes one essential part of a variable is easily obtainable from an automated database but another is not. For example, the number of vaginal births is available from most hospital databases; however, the percent of vaginal births that were V-backs (vaginal births following an earlier C-section) is more difficult to obtain because that information usually is not captured. Often individual services collect more detailed data about their specific cases, including outcomes, complications, and more extensive demographics.

With the growth in managed care programs and their impact on health care, the industry is experiencing increasing need for outcome data by physician, institution, and very specific diagnoses. More databases meeting these needs will evolve and hopefully will be organized to minimize duplication and maximize usefulness of the data.

Analyzing the Data and Using the Results to Make a Difference

The culmination of data collection is data analysis. The objective of data analysis is to provide accurate summary statistics and graphics that decision makers can use to make the most rational decisions possible. Because the objective of program evaluation is to define the results rather than to explain the process, there always is a chance that decisions are based on spurious results. In other words, the outcomes observed could be totally unrelated to the program and due to some other, unmeasured and unobserved factors. Thus, all data should be interpreted with caution, with the realization that causality is difficult if not impossible to demonstrate and that correlation may even be questionable.

Reports provided at the conclusion of a project should be clear, concise, and well organized. Presentation of data in table or chart form makes it easy to read. It also is important to follow good scientific principles in report writing and to ensure that the study design methodology and the data analysis procedures are well documented.

Graphs provide a very convenient and highly persuasive form of data display. Statistical packages for personal computers provide professional-looking graphs with a small investment of time spent in learning to use them. The presentation format should be planned based on the expected audience. Software packages available for personal computers allow anyone who can turn on a computer to prepare sophisticated, economical slides to augment every presentation.

It is important to try to identify where and when the evaluation program suffers from design flaws. Assumptions exist for every research project. If they do not hold (for example, the two groups were not matched on enough variables to define them as comparable), the problem should be publicly recognized. It is better that the program evaluator criticize his or her own work than to have someone else point out its weaknesses.

Finally, even though program evaluation is designed to make analysis of programs as objective as possible, it must be remembered that human organizations are not totally rational or objective systems. Although the research process and program evaluation are tools designed to maximize the likelihood that objective analysis and decisions can be made, the people making those decisions are still human beings and can and will act in spite of the best data. However, there is always room for improvement in the programs, as well as in the process of evaluation, each of which is a requisite for further study.

Recommendations for Making Care/Case Management Evaluation More Effective

Based on the experiences of a number of researchers, the following recommendations can be made to improve the effectiveness of care/case management program evaluation:

1. *Strive to include actual costs rather than charges or projections based on average costs and LOS reductions.* It is important to determine that practice changes are not increasing resource consumption while decreasing LOS, although it is recognized that cost data often are very difficult to obtain.

2. *Remember that all data have a price (the expense incurred in their collection).* This applies to cost data as well as to other types of data that are not easily accessible. It is important to balance the costs and benefits of obtaining different types of data, to make an informed decision about what is feasible given available resources, and to communicate decisions and rationales for these decisions, as well as results. If only a few indicators can be used, the evaluation of patients' clinical outcomes and cost per case should be considered the highest priorities. Outcomes such as patient and staff satisfaction are desirable to include but not as essential. (Some suggested tools for consideration in measuring these indicators are discussed at the conclusion of the section on quantitative data.)

3. *Begin to collect baseline data early.* This is important because the process of developing models and tools will create practice changes prior to full implementation and may result in underestimation of the effects of the program.

4. *Move toward evaluating long-term patient outcomes rather than focusing on primarily inpatient, episode-of-care discharge criteria.* Although evaluating long-term outcomes is likely to be more difficult and expensive, provider organizations cannot afford *not* to do it. Without this information, it will be extremely difficult to respond to payers' requests for the five-year survival rates for particular case types. Such requests are not uncommon in more fully developed managed care markets.

5. *Seek the assistance of a health economist or biostatistician in developing an analysis that considers and attempts to control for the effects of other factors*

on outcomes of interest. For example, Professor Robert Woodward of Washington University is working with the staff of Barnes Hospital in St. Louis in evaluating their Care Path program. He has analyzed their data using a multiple regression model that provides a basis for determining if outcomes for a case type population are significantly different after the introduction of Care Paths than what would have been expected based on previous trends.[21] Many forces affect LOS and cost, and this type of sophisticated analysis begins to provide a basis for causal inference, or at least establishes stronger links between care management implementation and decreased LOS and reduced cost. This is beyond the scope of program evaluation research comparing preimplementation and postimplementation averages. (Other key aspects of the comprehensive financial and clinical evaluation of Barnes's care management program are described by Weilitz and Potter.[22])

6. *Embed other types of research in the evaluation program.*[23] For example, Lamb[24] calls for research on the process of case management to define interventions in a way that connects process with outcomes. She points out that capitated systems prohibit the "shotgun" approach of doing everything and hoping something works. Instead, interventions need to be identified that effectively address causes of readmission amenable to case management, such as symptom control and access to care.

One approach to studying case manager practice would be to use the clinical narrative technique employed by Benner[25] to map the development of clinical nursing expertise. Williams[26] identifies the need to articulate the relationships between case management and nursing theory. Research on the process of nursing case management provides an opportunity for such an integration.

The following section discusses specific types of data and decisions required for the application of these principles and recommendations.

Categories of Data

Data can be defined as "our interpretation of recorded measurements or observations" and *observations* as "empirical evidence that we obtain in research."[27] There are two broad categories of data: qualitative and quantitative. As the names suggest, *qualitative* data have to do with the qualities or characteristics of a phenomenon, whereas *quantitative* data deal with quantities that can be measured. Thus, qualitative data are expressed in words, and quantitative data are represented by numbers.

Qualitative Data

Like all research, qualitative research basically is a process of formulating a question and gathering data to answer it. In this case, the question is one that can be answered appropriately with qualitative data.

Some of the most common techniques for collecting qualitative data include interviews, open-ended survey questions, and observation. *Interviews* are "conversations with a purpose,"[28] and they can be conducted with individuals or groups. Stephen and Kinsey[29] provide a relevant description of the use of different types of interviews and other types of data collection techniques for evaluating work redesign outcomes. In the context of evaluating the effects of implementing a care/case management program, it would be useful to interview, survey, and/or observe patients, staff nurses, case managers, and physicians.

The technique used to analyze qualitative data is called *content analysis* and is defined as "a procedure for the categorization of verbal or behavioral data, for purposes of classification, summarization and tabulation."[30] As the definition suggests, this process entails a careful review of the data to identify themes, the development of a set of categories, and the creation of a coding scheme for placing responses in categories. Usually the data are analyzed by two coders working independently to evaluate the consistency of their determinations (that is, reliability). One suggestion for decreasing the amount of work involved in processing the responses to open-ended questions is to ask respondents to help code their own answers.[31] For example, respondents can be asked to indicate if their comments are positive or negative. Sources of further information concerning qualitative data analysis include Glaser and Strauss[32] and Knafl and Webster.[33]

Schmitt and Klimoski[34] identify certain strengths and limitations of qualitative data. Following are the strengths of qualitative data:

- They are rich, full, holistic, and usually match the complexity of the phenomenon being studied.
- They can lead to serendipitous findings and new insights.

Following are the limitations of qualitative data:

- Collection and analysis are laborious and time-consuming.
- Methods of analysis are less well developed and thus the risk of drawing inappropriate inferences is somewhat higher.

Examples of Qualitative Evaluation

The literature on care/case management is filled with anecdotal accounts of the implementation of these programs in various facilities.[35] Descriptions or stories about what was done and how it was accomplished, accompanied by occasional unsubstantiated remarks that quality or satisfaction increased, are not examples of qualitative evaluation. The anecdotal approach can be very useful in sharing ideas with colleagues, especially when a concept is new, but it is not as complete as it could be. Before trying to adopt a new program, most organizations would prefer to have a clearer understanding of the effects it can produce. Given the development of care/case management in acute care over the past decade, it is time to move beyond descriptions of the implementation process and unconfirmed claims regarding outcomes.

A review of the literature revealed two particularly useful examples of care/case management evaluations that employed qualitative techniques. The first example was Van Dongen and Jambunathan's[36] pilot study of the role of the nurse case manager and perceived quality of care. This study incorporated data from participant responses to open-ended questions on a survey instrument. The authors surveyed 24 psychiatric outpatients, 5 registered nurse case managers (RNCMs), and 2 psychiatrists, and used the data obtained from these three groups to develop a composite description of RNCM care.

The questions to the patients included the following:

- How would you describe the care provided by your nurse in the outpatient department?
- What is most important to you about the care your nurse provides?
- What suggestions do you have for improving care?

Patients suggested that they "valued most the caring, supportive nature of the RNCM care provided." They differentiated the RNCM's role from the psychiatrist's role by describing the nurse as "more personable, accessible, and concerned with issues and problems of daily living beyond the psychiatric diagnoses and prescribed treatment. . . ."

The questions to the RNCMs included the following:

- What is most important in terms of your role?
- How do you perceive your role as different from other nursing roles you may have had in the past?
- What concerns do you have associated with your role as an RNCM?

RNCMs reported using the nursing process with "emphasis on general assessment, monitoring of medications, and supportive counseling" inherent in the nursing role. They characterized their role as "professional and independent, yet collaborative with the psychiatrist."

The questions to the psychiatrists included the following:

- What are your expectations for client care by the RNCM?
- What do you view as important in the care provided by the RNCM?
- What suggestions do you have for improving RNCMs' care?

Psychiatrists "valued the nurses for provision of ongoing management of care, monitoring of client condition, supportive counseling and education, and keeping the psychiatrist informed."

Although its findings are based on a small sample, this study examined interesting and important questions about a relatively new role and can serve as a basis for the development of further research.

The second example was the study by Collard, Bergman, and Henderson[37] in which a combination of qualitative and quantitative data was used to evaluate the care provided by medical case management programs (nurses managing cases for insurance companies). Data were gathered from two sources: (1) independent physician reviewer ratings of the appropriateness and adequacy of medical care, accompanied by narrative descriptions of their overall impressions of each case; and (2) client responses to structured interview questions concerning their attitudes toward and satisfaction with their case management program.

One component of this study involved interviews with 30 families of high-risk infants designed to answer three research questions. Following are the questions and their results:

1. *What services did parents of high-risk infants identify as arranged for by their case manager?* Parents identified services that frequently were arranged for by case managers (for example, case managers arranged for home care 60 percent of the time) but reported that services also were arranged for by others.
2. *What were the parents' attitudes toward case management?* Almost 75 percent of the parents indicated that they understood what medical case management was and that it met their expectations. Overall, 80 percent felt that the case manager was competent, professional, sensitive, and supportive. About one-third of the time parents were undecided and/or disagreed about 25 percent of the time as to whether case management provided their child with care that otherwise would not have been available or whether it coordinated their child's care better than they would have been able to themselves.
3. *Would parents of high-risk infants recommend case management to others in similar situations?* Forty percent strongly recommended case management, 3 percent did not recommend it, and more than half indicated that they "probably would" recommend it, "probably would not" recommend it, or "do not know" if they would recommend it.

The authors conclude that medical case management "can play an important role in maintaining high-quality medical care for critically ill patients and their families."

They note that the data suggest that the supportive, communicative role played by case managers is more important than service provisions, which points to the need for experienced, sympathetic health professionals in the case manager role.

The examples cited demonstrate the use of qualitative data in evaluating patient and caregiver outcomes. Patient satisfaction with services and willingness to recommend them to others also can be viewed as institutional outcomes. Thus, qualitative data could prove useful in evaluating an institution's reputation and image.

Quantitative Data

Quantitative data provide numeric measures of variables that reflect at least the frequency (the number of times an event occurred) and at most an exact measure of the amount of an occurrence.[38] According to Brink and Wood,[39] the distinguishing characteristic between qualitative and quantitative data is whether the data to be collected exist as, or can be converted into, numbers or whether they must remain verbal descriptions. Data that exist in the form of numbers or can be immediately transposed into numbers are considered quantitative.

Quantitative data are commonly described as one of four types depending on whether the data:

- Are put into a group (for example, sex and DRG are nominal variables)
- Fall into a ranked category (for example, patient classification categories and clinical ladder levels provide ordinal data)
- Represent a point on a continuum with equal distances between the points (interval data are exemplified by age, LOS, and cost)
- Have an absolute zero point (ratio data, such as temperature, weight, and length)

All quantitative data can be summarized by statistics.

In general, the hierarchical nature of the four types of data is considered when statistical summaries are planned. Although all common statistical procedures can be used with interval or ratio data, nominal data usually are summarized with frequencies, percentages, and contingency–correlation coefficients. Ordinal data also can use median, centiles, and rank-order coefficients.[40]

With all statistical analysis it is important to keep in mind that the outcomes of nonexperimental studies are suggestive and that any conclusions drawn from the analysis must be considered tentative until they can be replicated in a second or third, more rigorous (ideally experimental) research design.

Examples of Quantitative Evaluation

Objectives of care/case management programs generally can be evaluated using quantitative data. Cost and LOS are the most obvious and frequently reported variables in collaborative care studies. Both are *interval variables*. Patient and staff satisfaction often are measured with instruments that result in scores that are at least ordinal and, more likely, interval data. Less frequently reported variables include outcomes such as mortality, complications, readmission rates, staff turnover, and absenteeism. Depending on the focus of the study, specific outcome variables such as proportion of patients discharged home, time spent in intensive care units, and time spent intubated also will be reported. Although this chapter is not intended to be a comprehensive review of collaborative care studies, following are examples of study designs that demonstrate the use of quantitative measures.

Pretest and Posttest Design

In a replication of the Carondelet community-based model of nursing case management, Rogers, Riordan, and Swindle[41] quantify outcomes such as readmission rate,

LOS, net reimbursement, and system referrals. Their pretest and posttest design used similar time periods to gather comparative data on individual patients before and after they were entered into the case management program. Despite the assumption that chronic conditions would worsen over time and require more resources, in their early small sample (38 patients) the authors were able to demonstrate a 64 percent decrease in readmissions, a 50 percent decrease in LOS per admission, and an 80 percent decrease in overall costs.

In their study of the value of CareMaps for hip fracture patients, Ogilvie-Harris, Botsford, and Hawker[42] collected data on over 100 people divided into two groups. Their study was a pretest and posttest design with six months between measurements to train staff. In contrast to the Rogers and others study, this study involved different patients in the pretest group. The authors used several different quantitative measures, including ordinal scales measuring level of function and accommodation. Overall, patients in the study group had significantly better outcomes, including fewer postoperative complications and shorter LOS.

Comparison Group Design

Daly, Rudy, Thompson, and Happ[43] evaluated creation of a special care unit designed specifically to meet the needs of chronically critically ill patients. A physical design aimed at family involvement and rehabilitation, a shared governance management model, and a case management practice model were combined in a very innovative nurse-managed unit. This quasi-experimental design, involving randomly assigned patients in experimental or traditional units, provides good examples of quantitative evaluation measures. Demonstrated cost savings were related primarily to changes in nurse and physician staffing patterns, as well as to decreases in lab test utilization. Outcome measures for nurses included nurse satisfaction, and absenteeism and retention rates. Patient outcome measures included LOS, complications, mortality, readmission rate, and patient and family satisfaction with care. Although the initial article reported only preliminary findings about costs, the project appears well structured to provide comprehensive quantitative data.

Schull, Tosch, and Wood[44] studied the effectiveness of case managers for epilepsy patients by randomly assigning 42 patients to case-managed and non-case-managed groups. Although, overall, LOS was similar for both groups, a 26 percent decrease in LOS (1.97 days) was experienced among case-managed patients who were not undergoing seizure monitoring. Other variables studied included readmission rates, number of seizure-related emergency department visits, and ambulatory care clinic visits.

A third study of comparison groups randomly assigned patients to either an experimental case management or an existing system of care group to determine cost-effectiveness.[45] Although no real differences in cost, psychosocial adjustment, or quality of life scores were found, costs were shifted away from 24-hour and emergency care toward outpatient and case management services.

Combination Designs

In their study of the impact of major surgery critical paths on quality of care and cost, Shigemitsu and Tsushima[46] used a combination design involving comparison groups and pretest and posttest designs.

Patient satisfaction was measured via a survey distributed concurrently to study and comparison groups. In addition, long-term patient satisfaction was compared for pre- and post-managed-care patients by matching 35 study patients to patients treated the previous year. Variables of age, sex, LOS, and diagnosis-related group (DRG) were matched. One of the findings was that managed-care patients made fewer phone calls to the physician office between discharge and follow-up visit. Average LOS and charge comparisons also were favorable; however, comparisons across four DRGs in a total sample of only 35 patients prohibits conclusions until the sample can be increased.

Nurse/physician satisfaction was measured using a pretest/posttest design. A collaborative practice scale was distributed before implementation of the project and six months later. A high dropout rate of physician and nurse subjects occurred between the two time periods. As a result, only 25 percent of the original nurses were still in the sample at the second measurement. Thus, the nurse group was significantly changed. Although the average collaborative mean scores for nurse and physician increased in the postmeasurement period, the median test scores were not statistically different.

As part of Shigemitsu and Tsushima's study, nurse stress was measured before and after implementation of managed care. Results suggested that a significant increase in nurse job stress occurred following implementation of this care management program. Job stress was measured as the sum of 20 weighted statements about stressful events experienced during the previous day. As a result of this information, program administration was able to reevaluate problematic issues related to the following:

- The adequacy of staffing on each shift
- The availability of supervisory support for specific job skills
- The need to provide more praise for the staff

Although the study report is complicated, the evaluation design provides information about the expected outcomes and suggestions for follow-up studies that would provide further clarification. As a result of this study and the information obtained, evaluators and administrators are able to make program adjustments and revisions.

Further Methodological and Analytic Considerations for More Experienced Evaluators

The assumptions underlying statistical treatments need to be carefully adhered to whenever quantitative data are used. For example, most statistics rely on assumptions of normal distribution of data, that is, distributed under the familiar bell curve. Although experts urge that all data be reviewed to test assumptions of normality before performing sophisticated statistical analysis, this step is easily overlooked by evaluators.[47,48] If the data are skewed for any reason, special steps must be taken to match them to the statistic.

For example, during an evaluation of two types of programs (an experimental group and a control group) for treatment of rheumatoid arthritis, Sinacore, Chang, and Falconer[49] initially analyzed the data using variance analysis and concluded that there were no differences in the outcomes between the two programs. Subsequently, however, they discovered that the data did not meet the assumption of normal distribution required for this statistical test because the experimental group, who volunteered for the treatment being tested, were probably sicker than the control group. Reanalysis of the data using frequency histograms, which display results as a pattern of points on a graph, determined that the potentially sicker experimental group took significantly longer to demonstrate improvement. As a result of the nonnormal distribution, variance analysis could not reflect the true effects of the treatment and thus would have produced false conclusions. Use of frequency histograms to plot a point for each subject's result is an easy and visual way to examine the distribution of the data for normality.

Sometimes the most sophisticated statistics are not the best to use in summarizing data sets; on the other hand, restricting analysis of quantitative measures in program evaluation to simple statistics is not always an adequate alternative either. Most often, percent change or differences in means are used in the evaluation of care/case management programs. However, means are subject to distortion from outliers as well as nonnormal distributions. Keppel and Zedeck[50] recommend caution when using change scores, specifically the statistical difference between premeasures and postmeasures, to evaluate a program. They note that the change score usually is correlated with the premeasure or postmeasure score. Low premeasure scores will have greater difference scores than high premeasure scores. A second problem is that the difference score depends on the reliability of two measures. Thus, the difference score is less reliable than either of its components. The authors recommend using a hierarchical multiple regression strategy or an analysis of covariance to control for the problem. These analyses make it possible to determine what portion of the total effect is associated with the program and what portion is associated with the relationship between the change score and the measures.

Conclusion

When an organization implements a care/case management program, an evaluation plan must be developed to measure the program's benefits so that the organization can determine whether its investment in the program is worthwhile and whether its goals can be achieved. The process begins with development of a conceptual model and program objectives to give focus and structure to the evaluation plan. It is then important to consider the different research designs available for performing program evaluation. Program evaluation involves three basic components: (1) operationalizing the program's objectives, (2) selecting measurement tools to collect data, and (3) using the collected data to assess program outcomes and make changes as necessary.

Data obtained in the course of program evaluation fall into two broad categories: qualitative and quantitative. Qualitative data provide feedback expressed in words. Thus, these data can provide descriptions of patients' and caregivers' experiences and provide a rich source of information about issues such as satisfaction. Quantitative data provide statistical feedback that is useful in evaluating achievement of objectives related to variables such as length of stay or cost. Generally, most hospitals will include methods for obtaining both types of data in their evaluation plans to provide a comprehensive assessment of the outcomes of their collaborative care programs.

References

1. Collard, A. F., Bergman, A., and Henderson, M. Two approaches to measuring quality in medical case management programs. *Quality Review Bulletin* 16(1):3–8, 1990.

2. Shigemitsu, K., and Tsushima, G. Collaborative practice: nurse managed patient care. *SF Proceedings* 5(3):1–10, 1990.

3. Van Dongen, C. J., and Jambunathan, J. Pilot study results: the psychiatric RN case manager. *Journal of Psychosocial Nursing* 30(11):11–14, 1992.

4. Marks, B. A., and Hagenmueller, A. C. Technological and environmental characteristics of intensive care units: implications for job redesign. *Journal of Nursing Administration* 24(45):65–71, 1994.

5. Schmitt, N. W., and Klimoski, R. J. *Research Methods in Human Resources Management.* Cincinnati, OH: South-Western, 1991, p. 369.

6. Schmitt and Klimoski, p. 392.

7. Snyder, R. A., Raben, C. S., and Farr, J. L. A model for the systematic evaluation of human resource development programs. *Academy of Management Review* 5:433, 1980.

8. Schmitt and Klimoski.

9. Schmitt and Klimoski, p. 393.

10. Erkel, E. A. The impact of case management in preventive services. *Journal of Nursing Administration* 23(1):27–32, 1993.

11. Polit, D. F., and Hungler, B. *Nursing Research: Principles and Methods.* Philadelphia: Lippincott, 1991.

12. Wood, M. Evaluative designs. In: P. Brink and M. Wood, editors. *Advanced Design in Nursing Research.* Newbury Park, CA: Sage Publications, 1989, p. 223.

13. Wood, p. 225.

14. Shigemitsu and Tsushima, pp. 37–38.

15. Mishel, M. Methodological studies: instrument development. In: P. Brink and M. Wood, editors. *Advanced Design in Nursing Research.* Newbury Park, CA: Sage Publications, 1989.

16. National Institutes of Health. *Patient Outcomes Research: Effectiveness of Nursing Practice* (NIH Publication No. 93-3411). Rockville, MD: NIH, 1992.

17. Shigemitsu and Tsushima.

18. Weiss, S. J., and Davis, H. P. Validity and reliability of the collaborative practice scales. *Nursing Research* 34:299–305, 1982.

19. Kinzel, F. L. What's your stress level? *NurseLife* 2(2):54–55, 1982.

20. Isaac, S., and Michael, W. B. *Handbook in Research and Evaluation.* San Diego, CA: EDITS Publishers, 1981, p. 4.

21. Woodward, R. S. A comprehensive evaluation program at Barnes Hospital of St. Louis. Presented at The Center for Case Management Expert User Forum, San Antonio, Feb. 3, 1994.

22. Weilitz, P. B., and Potter, P. A. A managed care system: financial and clinical evaluation. *Journal of Nursing Administration* 23(11):51–57, 1993.

23. Stetler, C. Program evaluation: lessons learned. Presented at The Center for Case Management Expert User Forum, San Antonio, Feb. 4, 1994.

24. Lamb, G. Making a case for *nursing* case management. Presented at the Fifth National Conference on Nursing Administrative Research, Chapel Hill, NC, Oct. 15, 1993.

25. Benner, P. *From Novice to Expert: Excellence and Power in Clinical Nursing Practice.* Menlo Park, CA: Addison-Wesley, 1984.

26. Williams, B. S. The utility of nursing theory in nursing case management. *Nursing Administration Quarterly* 15(3):60–65, 1991.

27. Schmitt and Klimoski, p. 122.

28. Schmitt and Klimoski, p. 139.

29. Stephen, R. J., and Kinsey, M. G. A model for measuring outcomes of work redesign. In: K. J. McDonagh, editor. *Patient-Centered Care.* Ann Arbor, MI: Health Administration Press, 1993.

30. Fox, D. J. *Fundamentals of Research in Nursing.* New York City: Appleton-Century-Crofts, 1970, p. 262.

31. Schmitt and Klimoski.

32. Glaser, B. G., and Strauss, A. L. *The Discovery of Grounded Theory: Strategies for Qualitative Research.* New York City: Aldine, 1967.

33. Knafl, K., and Webster, D. Managing and analyzing qualitative data: a description of tasks, techniques, and materials. *Western Journal of Nursing Research* 110:195–218, 1988.

34. Schmitt and Klimoski, pp. 151–52.

35. Marschke, P., and Nolan, M. T. Research related to case management. *Nursing Administration Quarterly* 17(3):16–21, 1993.

36. Van Dongen and Jambunathan.

37. Collard and others.

38. Brink, P., and Wood, M. *Advanced Design in Nursing Research.* Newbury Park, CA: Sage Publications, 1989, p. 13.

39. Brink and Wood, p. 12.

40. Waltz, C., Strickland, O., and Lenz, E. *Measurement in Nursing Research.* Philadelphia: F. A. Davis Company, 1984.

41. Rogers, M., Riordan, J., and Swindle, D. Community-based nursing case management pays off. *Nursing Management* 22(3):30–34, 1991.

42. Ogilvie-Harris, D., Botsford, D., and Hawker, R. Elderly patients with hip fractures: improved outcome with the use of care maps with high-quality medical and nursing protocols. *Journal of Orthopaedic Trauma* 7(5):428–37, 1993.

43. Daly, B., Rudy, E., Thompson, K., and Happ, M. Development of a special care unit for chronically critically ill patients. *Heart & Lung* 20(1):45–51, 1991.

44. Schull, D., Tosch, P., and Wood, M. Clinical nurse specialists as collaborative care managers. *Nursing Management* 23(3):30–33, 1993.

45. Jerrell, J., and Hu, T. Cost-effectiveness of intensive clinical and case management compared with an existing system of care. *Inquiry* 26:224–34, Summer 1989.

46. Shigemitsu and Tsushima.

47. Polit and Hungler.

48. Shelley, S. I. *Research Methods in Nursing and Health*. Boston: Little, Brown and Company, 1984.

49. Sinacore, J., Chang, R., and Falconer, J. Seeing the forest despite the trees. *Evaluation and the Health Professions* 15(2):131–46, 1992.

50. Keppel, G., and Zedeck, S. *Data Analysis for Research Design*. New York City: Witt Freeman & Co., 1989.

CHAPTER TEN

A Look to the Future

Karen Zander

Today's providers of direct care are faced with a dilemma that Annas[1] succinctly noted a few years ago in an article in *The Boston Globe:* "The three major issues confronting us are, of course, cost, quality, and access. The policy problem we have consistently refused to acknowledge is that all three of these issues must be dealt with simultaneously. Dealing with only one at a time will ultimately be self-defeating." Collaborative care via CareMap systems and case management — and the strategies that have evolved from them — is an attempt to address these major issues at the client–provider level. It produces synergistic effects that transform patterns of utilization within the health care institution, which is being responded to by administrators who possess both social conscience and business acumen. Contemporary solutions lie in collaboratively determined answers such as the ones described throughout this text.

Using CareMap tools around the clock for the management and evaluation of outcome-driven care by all disciplines constitutes a system of collaborative outcomes management. Through the well-established process of assessment and the new process of variance analysis, care is individualized and any necessary corrective actions are begun in a timely, coordinated manner. In addition, variances can be trended and aggregated as data for continuous quality improvement (CQI) endeavors. Organizations that have fully integrated their CareMap document into their documentation system have overcome a variety of obstacles and are beginning to make knowledgeable decisions using on-line, clinician-generated data. Integration of the CareMap document will enable these organizations to restructure operations with good information and, hopefully, wisdom.

Organizations using case managers as the coordinators or expediters of care also are experiencing positive results. Because case management "is a major departure from the way we have organized work since the Industrial Revolution,"[2] intense comparative evaluations and precision design of models will be needed over the next few years.

This chapter looks at the future of health care by studying two changes in collaborative care that will be imperative to its survival. These are (1) automation of the multidisciplinary clinical record so that the outcome-based CareMap tool drives the entire information network and (2) accountability structures within disciplines, both at a matrix level and on the larger care continuum.

Automation of the Clinical Record

The first fundamental element of future collaborative care strategies is automation of the CareMap tool. Currently, the CareMap tool component of collaborative care is paper dependent. Although some paper CareMap tools are quite sophisticated and even artful, all are limited by the two-dimensionality of the paper itself as well as by practical problems such as storage. The entire benefit of a CareMap system cannot be realized until it has all the access, three-dimensionality (depth), and breadth of linkages that automation can provide.

Although the people in collaborative care can go a long way toward creating a nonfragmented care delivery system, the process of care delivery depends on information, and currently information on every aspect of patient care is immensely fragmented. The problem is only compounded by the tendency of organizations to create and/or purchase a new stand-alone automated system for every new data need, rather than demand integration before purchasing an automated product.

The rationale for an automated CareMap system goes far beyond ease of documentation and access of information for the direct caregiver. In *Making Managed Healthcare Work*, Boland describes a set of 12 requirements to truly enable a health care network of organizations to manage care. These 12 requirements include everything from capital to a full array of health care services. Of the 12 building blocks of Boland's proposed third-generation delivery system,[3] at least 5 could be addressed through an automated CareMap system:

1. Communications
2. Utilization management
3. Quality
4. Reporting
5. Information

For information systems alone, Boland describes a number of characteristics. These include:

- Routine integration of inpatient and ambulatory data with performance indicators on quality, efficiency, and cost
- Ad hoc inquiry into relationships between financial, clinical, and utilization data
- On-line modeling of alternative treatment plans
- Multiple software modules running simultaneously to access data from different delivery system functions

Potential of Automated CareMap Tools

Because a CareMap tool visually shows a standardized and relational schedule of process, outcome, and variance, each requiring a yes–no response as well as the capability of scripted responses, it lends itself well to automation. Indeed, CareMap tools originally were designed with automation in mind. What has evolved since their inception is the amount of functionality possible through their use.

For example, automation would facilitate accurate care planning by merging two or more CareMap tools, allowing the clinician to see and recall relationships between procedures, comorbidities, and stage/phase of illness. Even more important, automation would assist the clinician in either adapting standard CareMap tools for individual needs or building completely new maps "from scratch." When more is known about the best practices that lead to outcomes and predictor modeling, it will be possible to improve assessments themselves and, based on certain assessment data, the computer might suggest varieties of maps.

The task completion and the intermediate or final outcome achievement criteria outlined on the CareMap tool should become the computer transactions that (1) lead the clinician to further actions or information and (2) automatically record the transaction for further aggregating and analysis. For example, when a physical therapist validates that a patient's range of motion has met a specific degree, the physical therapy note is automatically printed for that patient *and* the computer can store range-of-motion measurements for all similar patients. However, if the physical therapist confirms that the patient has not been able to achieve that range of motion, the therapist is automatically led to a variance analysis screen. At this point, the therapist needs to address three questions:

1. What is the actual-versus-planned range of motion?
2. Why has the planned range of motion not been met?
3. What corrective action should be initiated?

To explore why the planned range of motion has not been met, the therapist should code (categorize) the question according to cause, such as too much pain, and send it via the computer to be documented as a progress note and a variance for further study. The payer may also need to know the therapist's assessment of the patient's condition to understand subsequent treatment and discharge decisions. To consider corrective actions that will answer the questions, the therapist should call up a prompter list of suggestions and an array of options and specialists, one of whom might function as an immediate "consultant." The computer also might let the therapist know of current organizational/regional/national statistics or research used to correct similar situations.

At the same time, the computer can charge for the physical therapy visit because the therapist is interacting with it. The therapist could be doing this documentation from the bedside, the unit station, the home visit, or the office. In fact, any department can be given schedules in advance if a CareMap tool is used for resource scheduling on admission. In addition, individual time management tools might be generated per day for physicians, nurses, and professionals from other disciplines who need to deliver direct service.

As all disciplines and departments record their transactions, advanced information systems could calculate total patient acuity or intensity, as well as actual, comprehensive costs in acute care and beyond (for example, home health, long-term care, primary care, and community services). In this way, true costs can be captured and managed. Barrett describes the next logical step:

Managed Care and capped reimbursement will increasingly become the typical reimbursement method making cost the only alternative for increasing profit margins. Improving the efficiency of patient care, as a result, may be the most significant opportunity for cost reductions. Such improvements can be implemented while maintaining or improving the quality of care—if adequate tools are available.[4]

When a whole group of similar patients (such as cardiology patients) is managed and the care delivered by all disciplines is automatically evaluated for quality and costed for resource use or changes in staffing mix or technology, care processes can be evaluated more objectively over time. Additionally, a few institutions are experimenting with using maps to perform other functions—for example, to anticipate materials management needs, anticipate patient care assignments to nursing staff by day, or define specific research criteria as to either the processes of care or specific patient/family responses to care. Obviously, these functions and more will be exponentially enhanced with an automated relational database.

Laying the Groundwork for Automation

Weilitz[5] describes three phases of paper CareMap development: current practice, best practice, and ideal practice. *Current practice* occurs when actual practice is authored on a paper document to test in practice and revise. Current practice CareMaps are preliminary documents that help an author team converse and collaboratively question their own processes and outcomes. *Best practice* occurs when maps are written as a second version once the author team's members review their own discipline's standards and professional literature. *Ideal practice* occurs when the author team and others from their departments/services begin to benchmark various aspects of, and data from, practice with other organizations. This process may take a year or more, after which the author team or collaborative group incorporates new processes into practice and onto their maps.

At the current slow rate of automation and integration of information, it is likely that most institutions will have best-practice maps on paper by the time they are ready for automation and benchmarking. The following suggestions may help lay the groundwork for automation:[6]

1. *Perfect the paper:* By developing manual CareMap systems first, clinicians will better understand the patterns, process, and costs associated with care.
2. *Be brief:* Narrative notes should be eliminated because long stories do not lend themselves to either computerized documentation or mapping. Codes should be developed and statements should be short and concise.
3. *Define the product:* Clinicians should know what they want before shopping for software vendors. They should be prepared to ask vendors about their plans for integrating with other systems, managing multiple maps for patients with comorbidities, and so on.
4. *Think beyond paper:* Automated systems will not be useful if they are designed to simply show a paper system on a terminal. Automation must be able to provide all the background information clinicians need to deliver high-quality health care.
5. *Develop spreadsheets:* Although spreadsheets are two-dimensional software, they are a necessary step in developing the data generated from mapping systems because they can provide information for discerning patterns and making decisions.
6. *Integrate:* It is important to ensure that any clinical software integrates with existing financial, order-entry, or admission software. The health care industry is moving toward a community health integrated network, which requires the marriage of clinical and financial information.

Figure 10-1 shows the flow from current paper practice to automated ideal practice, which for most institutions will be the time at which the information systems (I/S) vendors will have products that integrate information necessary for the efficient management of care. As shown, one large impetus for integrated information and clinical management systems will be the payer changes.

Pending Issues

Although automation of a CareMap system seems a natural next step, it may raise as many questions as it resolves. For example, format across an institution, and even a community, may have to be standardized before everyone is in agreement. In addition to format, other pending issues include validity and reliability of patterns and outcome verification, access, and conceptualization of the work itself. In fact, the unresolved conflicts of collaborative care will most likely be fought and resolved within

Figure 10-1. Evolution from Current Practice to Automated Ideal Practice

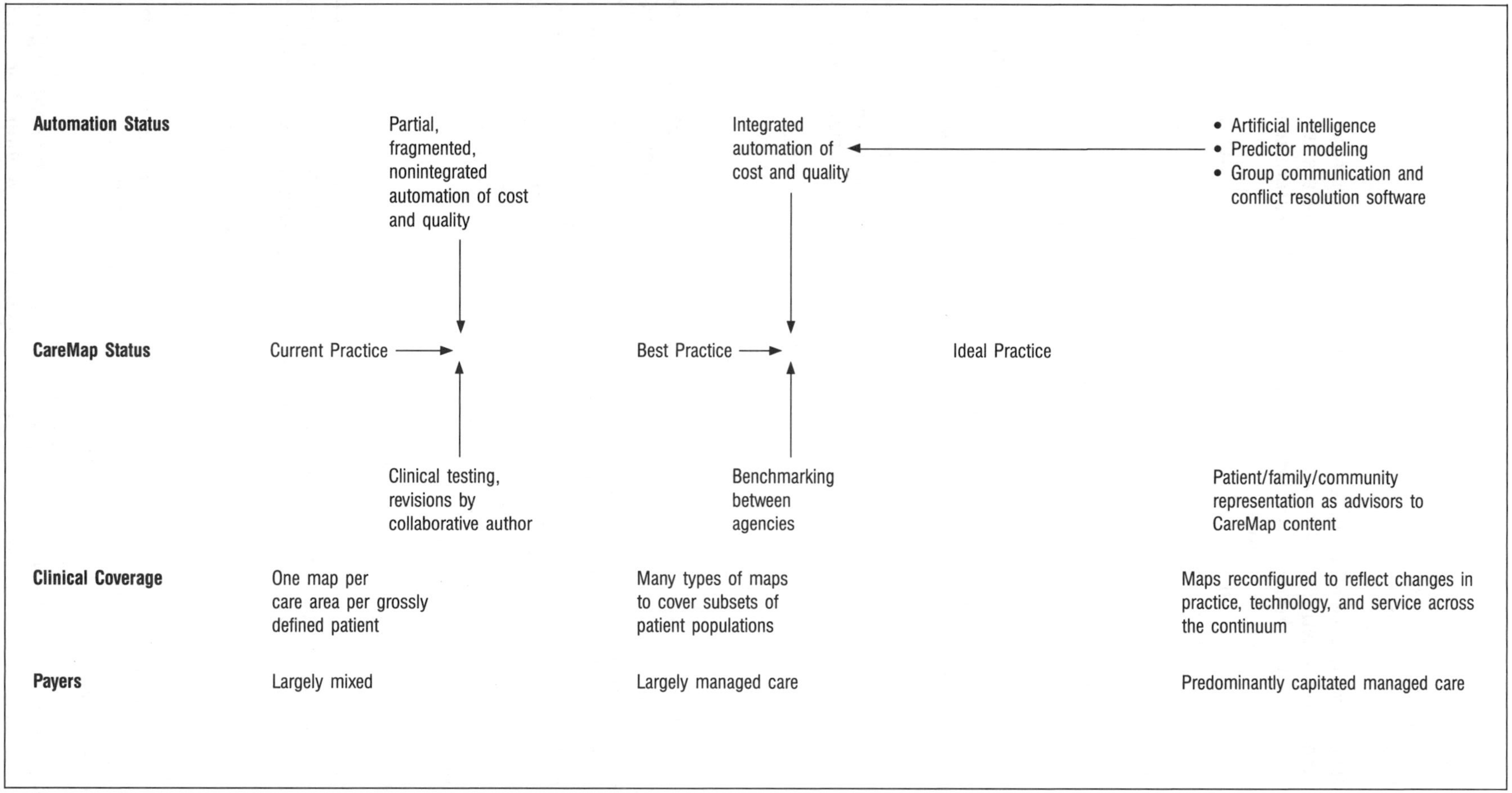

	Current Practice →	Best Practice →	Ideal Practice
Automation Status	Partial, fragmented, nonintegrated automation of cost and quality	Integrated automation of cost and quality	• Artificial intelligence • Predictor modeling • Group communication and conflict resolution software
CareMap Status	Clinical testing, revisions by collaborative author	Benchmarking between agencies	Patient/family/community representation as advisors to CareMap content
Clinical Coverage	One map per care area per grossly defined patient	Many types of maps to cover subsets of patient populations	Maps reconfigured to reflect changes in practice, technology, and service across the continuum
Payers	Largely mixed	Largely managed care	Predominantly capitated managed care

the intellectual arena of software content and logic. In other words, power struggles over access to data, control of algorithms, outcome language, and other kinds of information will emerge as new software is designed and selected.

There are a number of ways to avoid unnecessary conflict when automating each discipline's CareMap content and processes. For example:

- The urge to have all processes standardized should be resisted until the cause-and-effect relationships between processes and results are understood.
- A common language—with definitions—should be established between disciplines whenever possible.
- Former patients and their families should be included as advisors in the validation of language and timing of outcomes.
- I/S vendors should be selected who can easily link information for all users.
- The same steering committee involved from the beginning should be maintained throughout the automation implementation.
- Learning how to benchmark successfully should be achieved. (The Joint Commission on Accreditation of Healthcare Organizations[7] is a good resource for benchmarking models.)
- All data should be returned to the original author teams for review.
- An agencywide mechanism should be established for education and quality control and improvement of the automated clinical CareMap system.

Even when CareMap tools become more sophisticated and ultimately automated, in themselves they will not tell an organization how to structure itself. A CareMap system describes outcome-based practice in theory; it is the clinicians who make it come alive for each patient and family.

Structures for Accountability

The second fundamental element of future collaborative care strategies is strengthening operational structures for outcome accountability. In other words, unless the care delivery organization establishes a better infrastructure for accountability for outcomes than currently exists, payers and other business groups will more aggressively insert themselves into the content and process of care delivery. More important, unclear or absent accountability structures can produce confusion and regression among caregivers, resulting at times in lack of clinical precision and nonoptimal clinical outcomes. There needs to be accountability within each discipline, both at the matrix level and on a larger continuum.

Current Accountability Status

Accountability is the answerability for the outcomes or results of one's work. It implies and assumes that the authority necessary to act or intervene has been acquired. In fact, accountability is the highest phase of professional growth and role development, which begins with knowledge, skills, and values; builds with responsibilities; and matures with authority,[8] as illustrated by the following progression:

Knowledge, skills, values ⟶ Responsibility ⟶ Authority ⟶ Accountability

Often clinicians are caught in a maze of ambiguous accountability, which impedes collaboration and threatens potential patient and family outcomes. This mire might be characterized by the following conditions:

- *Each discipline has only partial knowledge of the skill for, and value of, collaboration.* Collaboration is not a formal component of the clinical education of caregivers. Because collaboration often involves more time and different skills than direct clinical expertise, it is not practiced as automatically as it should be. Because it is not practiced, it receives lower status and is not valued as much as technical prowess.

- *Multiple and often overlapping responsibilities exist between departments and disciplines.* This confusing condition could get worse if an organization puts all its restructuring efforts into shifting tasks rather than restructuring the next level—authority.
- *Authority to act is unclear in the care-giving arena.* The traditional model that any and all authority stems solely from physician orders is inaccurate and inefficient. For example, transferring patients out of an ICU to a floor can be problematic because the authority for the decision is vague. Even if the transfer criteria are clear, getting the decision made can take one to two days even with uncomplicated patients.
- *Members of nonmedical disciplines ultimately default accountability to physicians.* This is true especially when collaborative assessment and planning are perceived as impossible. Clarification and evaluation of outcomes achievable for each patient and family have been handled sporadically. The most collaborative review of outcomes has tended to be in the rehabilitation and psychiatric settings, but even there clinicians can become frustrated with each other when trying to make timely, practiced decisions.

Currently, the clinicians do not have the cost and quality data, the administrative people who do have the data do not know how to evaluate it without clinician input, and the whole care-giving organization is legally accountable for outcomes even though payers are attempting to make clinical decisions. Thus, the question is: Where to start to build accountability? The answer is that accountability should be built from the patient/family's care and outcomes upward and outward.

If hospitals are to be truly patient focused, they must structure accountability for patient outcomes at one if not two levels. These are:[9]

1. *The care management level* (that is, within a unit or area of care): At The Center for Case Management, it is believed that 100 percent of patients need their care managed via CareMap tools wherever possible and via formal accountability methods.
2. *The case management level:* The Center also believes that it is crucial that a smaller number of patients, possibly 20 percent, have case managers in addition to, or possibly instead of, a CareMap system.

Accountability at the care delivery level entails answerability for clinical outcomes, whereas accountability at the case management level includes answering for overall financial outcomes as well as short- and long-range clinical outcomes. At both levels, the clinical outcomes should be those that are important to patients/families as well as to care providers and their organizations.

It must be noted that accountability is more than an attitude. It must be built into a role, a job description, and a formal evaluation process. Until recently, accountability for health care professionals other than physicians has been rather loosely defined, left to the motivation of each individual and the interpretation of immediate supervisors. On the other hand, physicians are held accountable for outcomes such as mortality, morbidity, and infection rates—a purely negative, regulatory approach. Neither kind of accountability—loose or regulatory—is ideal. Thus, new definitions are necessary.

Now that an agency's livelihood is contingent on both sound clinical and financial management, achieving patient/family outcomes of care is paramount. Because cost and quality — as measured by tangible outcomes rather than solely satisfaction levels — are being monitored ever more vigilantly by diverse internal and external groups, the "age of accountability" is here.

Accountability at the Care Management Level

As discussed previously in this book, all professional groups including physicians, social workers, physical therapists, and so on are rethinking their accountabilities. At the shift and unit levels, these disciplines are working with nursing in attempts to stabilize the services they provide. Because these levels have so many implications for nursing, nursing departments currently are evaluating their internal, unit-based structures for accountability. Currently, nursing has three choices at the care delivery level: (1) no accountability, in which nurse managers are accountable but so bogged down with other responsibilities that accountability ultimately defaults to the physician; (2) primary nursing, in which every eligible nurse is required to function for patients/families beyond the completion of tasks on a shift; and (3) care management (care co-ordination), in which nurses functioning similarly to primary nurses are assigned by unit district or, more often, case type, physician, or some other definer. (See chapter 1 for more detailed discussion of these three options.)

Accountability at the Case Management Level

As mentioned previously, case management is *not* a care delivery system and its design should not be determined exclusively by one department. There are two principal models for structuring accountability via case management: clinical nursing and utilization review (UR). (For a more complete discussion of case management structures for accountability, see chapter 1.)

Despite their similar appearance, the clinical nursing and UR models have very different assumptions underlying their use. Although both have management of the cost per case budget as a major responsibility, how the cost and clinical outcomes per case are actually negotiated within a network of services is quite different. (See figure 10-2.)

Presently, hospitals are experimenting with combining UR, discharge planning, and, at times, social service under one case management umbrella. In this design, all patient conditions would be reviewed via the medical record as they are now and, in addition, those patients requiring more extensive discharge planning would be interviewed directly and an appropriate plan devised. The main difference between clinical and the more administrative case management role just described is authority for day-to-day problem solving that may have nothing to do with discharge planning. Clinical case managers tend to get actively involved in problem solving with the direct caregivers. Both models require collaborative skills, may be formally linked to individual or group physician practices, and are a means for defining accountability.

A case manager's success depends on the skill and energy of the individuals providing direct service from all departments. This fact raises three fundamental questions:

1. How can accountability for cost and quality outcomes be kept as close as possible to the direct caregivers?
2. How can new shifts in authority between disciplines be negotiated and supported within a collaborative environment?
3. How can a whole organization be structured so that accountabilities are as clear as possible?

What is emerging are two levels of outcome accountability — one for the cost and clinical outcomes per discipline per patient/family as described precisely on CareMap tools or more reflectively in the traditional chart, and another for cost and clinical outcomes for groups of patients/families per service, product line, center of excellence, and so on. If this evolution continues, structures for accountability will be formed within the context of a matrix organization.

The Matrix Structure

The challenges of maintaining professional autonomy within a collaborative milieu and departmental sanctity while trying to attain the common good of the whole can best be met by a matrix structure. A *matrix* is a "multiple command system with related support mechanisms and associated culture and behavior patterns in complex organizations which have outside pressure for dual focus, high information-processing capacity, and pressures for shared resources."[10]

Figure 10-2.   Comparison of Case Management Profiles: Utilization Review and Clinical Nursing Departments

	UR/UM Case Management	Clinical Case Management
Why?	Concurrent and retrospective review of care to determine appropriate setting. Focus is on payer and justification of care, length of stay, and interventions. Concern is with appropriateness and efficiency.	Coordinate, advocate, and expedite care, especially care of complex and catastrophic illness across multiple care settings, including beyond acute care into community. Concern is with efficiency and producing measurable clinical outcomes. Model may include a prevention/ health maintenance focus.
Who?	RNs from diverse educational backgrounds	RNs from diverse educational backgrounds depending on model
What?	UR/UM conducts 100% review of appropriate setting for patient care. May include: • Risk management • Discharge planning • Caseload is 20–25 patients per day	• Case managers usually manage approximately 20% of a total acute care population to provide continuity of both care plan and direct care providers or teams. • Caseload varies from 1–200 based on model design.
Where?	May be assigned by payer; UM tends to be assigned by service.	May be assigned by: • Diagnosis or procedure • Age • Insurer • Service • Product line • Community residence • If assigned by unit, etc., is considered care manager
When?	Daily review	Daily review when a case manager is on duty; if a CareMap system is in place, reviews variances from CareMap tool that occurred during absence in order to understand and facilitate. A few case management models have 7-day/week coverage.
How?	Primarily chart review using nationally accepted review standards	Working with and through all departments and disciplines by: (1) use of a clinical reasoning and problem-solving process, and (2) creating, maintaining, and negotiating a network of services.

Case Management and the Matrix Structure

In whole and in each of its component parts, collaborative care is in effect synonymous with matrix. The CareMap tool is itself a multicommand document, and case management definitely represents the integration of multiple work processes and resources. In fact, like matrix, case management cuts across the functional divisions of labor. "In general, organizations with complex processes for bringing their products and services to market are the best candidates for case management. . . . In creating case management environments, the firms we studied faced several issues. Managers must deal with such implementation issues as the proximity of the case manager to the customer, the decision rights granted to case managers, the supporting information architecture, the level of monitoring, and the choice between individuals and teams as case managers."[11]

At present, hospitals, home care, and many outpatient services are experimenting with case management but have not significantly restructured administration to support it. Rather, they have paid more attention to restructuring levels below or parallel to the case manager. However, going by the definition that case managers manage processes rather than people, it would make more sense to concentrate efforts on levels above the case manager. If the people in upper-management roles, such as the vice-president of patient care services and the vice-president of quality management, cannot agree on priorities and goals, the relatively fragile beginnings of case management will not be vigorously supported or honestly evaluated. In fact, an organization may unknowingly fall victim to one or more "matrix pathologies" such as excessive overhead, decision strangulation, layering (matrixes within matrixes), and power struggles.[12]

Because case managers are self-managing, they do not need intense supervision. However, they would benefit from assistance in the areas of secretarial support, open access to information, and routine clarification of boundaries and goals. They also would require peer consultation within their own groups.[13]

Although at present case managers usually are paid by one of three departments (nursing, utilization management, or physicians), their future reporting mechanism will most likely be the product line or center of excellence. A separate department of case management may be an interim step, but it has the disadvantage of pigeonholing what should be a dynamic, linking-pin function.

Product Lines and the Matrix Structure

Ultimately, product lines or centers of excellence will cross care settings as much as possible, controlling a capitation budget. This expansion would include all forms of outpatient care as well as support groups, wellness programs, hospice, and long-term care. Each managed care/product line may be codirected by an institutional representative and a formally appointed physician, with data support provided by an information specialist. The number and type of case managers necessary to expedite care, once most patients have automated CareMap tools and other episodic services in place, will be determined by the product line administration.

Donovan and Matson[14] predict that the 1990s will be "the decade to confront outpatient care" because of a shift of 30 to 40 percent of traditional admissions from inpatient to outpatient settings. They cite these three trends:

1. Changing patient demographics
2. Stricter payer initiatives
3. Technological advances

With the advent of many creative new services in multiple sites, each with its own array of clinical experts, the service or product line version of matrix management increasingly will be the structure of choice. For example, the administrative structure of a center of excellence in oncology can provide a variety of services, both inpatient and outpatient, including case management, working within each patient's "budget." With automation, these centers will have the data to continue to make timely, responsive decisions as clinical practice becomes more collaborative and sophisticated.

Smaller Institutions and the Matrix Structure

Smaller institutions having very diverse patient populations with only a few admissions in each "category" may not need centers of excellence as such. However, collaborative practice and collaborative administrative teams still will be essential to the provision of services by smaller institutions.

Often a region's sole health care provider, a smaller institution will need a matrix organization to develop collaborative care strategies for a fluid work force. As formal teams of physicians, nurses, pharmacists, physical therapists, dietitians, social workers, and others begin to span an episode and eventually a continuum of care, they will need an equally flexible and far-reaching administration.

An example of the early phases of this phenomenon can be found at Good Samaritan Hospital in Lebanon, Pennsylvania. Thirty percent of the nursing staff (RNs and eventually LPNs and aides) are educated to be utilized between the hospital and home care. Community physicians already treat patients in both arenas and presently are being assisted by the hospital pharmacy and other departments. The hospital's innovations are summarized below:[15]

- In obstetrics, teams of nurses make prenatal house calls, follow patients through delivery, and handle in-home postpartum checkups to teach new mothers breast feeding and other tasks. The arrangement has helped ease insurers' restrictions on length of stay (LOS), which were constraining the amount of postpartum education.
- Stabilized patients with end-stage heart disease are being released home, with visits by critical care nurses who have trained family caregivers to assist with dobutamine drips. Care is guided by protocols developed with cardiologists on staff.
- In partnership with nearby Philhaven Hospital in Mount Giefna, Pennsylvania, psychiatric nurses are trained in home care procedures to handle pre-admission and postdischarge care, reducing waiting times and eventual LOS. Through Philhaven's inpatient programs, Good Samaritan home care patients showing signs of depression can be referred for a home visit from one of the psychiatric nurses from Philhaven.

By being both profitable and collaborative, Good Samaritan Hospital has been able to continuously adjust its work force to its census without resorting to layoffs. CareMap systems will facilitate their care giving between hospital and home. However, their model is not case management but, rather, a new care delivery approach. Good Samaritan and similar pioneering institutions should be observed over time to study how the transformation of services at the patient–clinician level causes other necessary transformations in information and administrative support activities.

Educational Preparation and Differentiation

As described previously in this text, collaborative care is a type of care engaged in by professional clinicians to enable them to be accountable for outcomes. Obviously, the background for outcome-based practice must be provided in each discipline's formal education process (see chapter 4 for in-service training on the use of CareMaps).

More case examples, simulations for experiential learning, and actual team-building curricula all will be needed. Ideally, professional schools might build a course that offered a health care team–guided experience.

Clinicians would be greatly encouraged to conduct care accountably and collaboratively if they saw that administrators conducted themselves accountably and collaboratively. (Clinicians particularly focus on the way the chief executive officer handles relationships with and between the vice-president of patient services, finance, and physicians.) Otherwise, the skills and attitudes gained by clinicians eventually will be dropped if they find themselves working in an organization that does not value those behaviors. Certainly, continuous quality improvement (CQI) education for administrators has made a positive difference in many organizations. The initial momentum that CQI created should be augmented at this time by (1) learning about matrix management before restructuring and (2) investing in good team functioning "at the top."

Clinicians grappling with the meaning of outcomes to their practice will pursue several related subject areas. In addition to keeping current with the latest findings, medications, and technology in their respective fields, they will benefit from revisiting some of the "classics." These include:

- Epidemiology
- Statistics
- Functional health patterns
- Nutrition
- Patient education techniques
- Dealing with psychological impact of the crisis of illness

They also may want to know more about care settings and treatment techniques outside their own domain. For example:

- Long-term care
- Wellness clinics
- Acupuncture, chiropractic
- Holistic healing

Along with the new skills and knowledge about producing outcomes will come more confidence and clarity in the kinds of outcomes for which clinicians will be willing to be accountable. As this redefinition proceeds, two trends will emerge: First, outcomes for which the patient/family are accountable or need to be more active in achieving (for example, smoking cessation) will be clear and may even take the form of treatment contracts common now in psychiatric programs. Second, clinicians will begin to self-select the level of outcome and scope of practice within which they are most comfortable working. Ideally, there will be an array of very specific positions from which a professional may choose, each outlining the nature of clinical and financial outcomes expected.

Educators will definitely be scrambling to offer viable programs at basic and advanced levels in each discipline. They might consider entering into a collaborative practice with health care consultants so that the strengths of both "supporting roles" in the field today can be available to organizations undergoing pressures not experienced until recently.

Conclusion

In the future, collaborative care via strategies such as CareMap tools and case management will stimulate many natural transitions in the way health care is delivered. From

the present perspective, a number of these transitions can be predicted with some cer
tainty. For example, CareMap documents will likely be automated and integrated into
the organization's documentation system. Additionally, clinical interactions will drive
all related patient care information such as cost, acuity, and scheduling.

Nursing will provide accountability at the unit level via primary nursing or care
coordinators. Case managers, either clinical or administrative, will be used widely to
integrate care-giving processes within and between organizations. Eventually, organizations will choose formal matrix structures at the product line/center of excellence
level and, ultimately, case managers will report to that level.

Administrators will need to function more collaboratively if they expect professional clinicians to do the same. As for clinicians, formal academic professional schools
will have to mobilize quickly to prepare new and advanced clinicians for the behaviors
required by collaborative care, and even the most traditional practitioners may begin
to learn more about healing and wellness as payment methods cover a continuum of
care.

Collaborative care is effective because it occurs where the real action takes place
and where all analyses should begin and end. It is easy to become overwhelmed by
or sidetracked from this primary activity. At the heart of care delivery redesign must
be the individual patient and family and their clinical outcomes. Otherwise, the purpose of the work will be lost.

Changes that either are too elaborate or detract from the ultimate importance of
clinical care will undermine any larger, loftier enterprise. Organizations that embrace
the culture and methods of collaborative care will meet their mission to society as
they seek new ways to deliver efficient and effective care.

References

1. Annas, G. Rationing health care. *The Boston Globe*, July 22, 1990, p. A-1.

2. Davenport, T., and Nohria, N. Case management and the integration of labor. *Sloan Management Review* 35(2):14,16, Winter 1994.

3. Boland, P. *Making Managed Healthcare Work.* Rockville, MD: Aspen, 1993, pp. 541–42.

4. Barrett, M. Continuum-of-care case management. *Computers in Healthcare* 14(8):25, June 1993.

5. Weilitz, P. Presentation during Fast-tracking CareMap System and Case Management Implementation Conference, St. Louis, MO, Aug. 1, 1993.

6. Tackbary, M. T., and Bean, B. Untitled. Planned for publication in Mar. 1995. Health Management
   Technology.

7. Joint Commission on Accreditation of Healthcare Organizations. Benchmarking in health care: models
   for improvement. *Journal on Quality Improvement* 20(5), May 1994.

8. Bergman, R. Accountability: definition and dimensions. *International Nursing Review* 28(2):53–59,
   Mar.–Apr. 1991.

9. Zander, K. Case management series, part I. *The New Definition* 9(2):1–2, Spring 1994.

10. Davis, S., and Lawrence, P. *Matrix.* Reading, MA: Addison-Wesley Publishing Co., 1977.

11. Davenport and Nohria, p. 16.

12. Davis and Lawrence.

13. Shields, J., and others. *Peer Consultation in the Group Context.* New York City: Springer Publishing,
    1985.

14. Donovan, M., and Matson, T., editors. *Outpatient Case Management.* Chicago: American Hospital
    Publishing, 1994, p. 7.

15. Lumsden, K. It's a jungle out there! *Hospitals and Health Networks* 68(10):65, May 20, 1994.

Additional Books of Interest

An Executive Guide to Case Management Strategies
by Marjorie A. Satinsky, MBA, FACHE
copublished with the New England Healthcare Assembly

This book describes how to plan, organize, develop, and improve case management programs so that they reach their full potential in the clinical and financial management of care. Readers will be able to make programs more effective across care settings and integrated delivery networks by utilizing the planning framework outlined in the book and the practical advice provided in the five case studies. Chief operating officers, nurse executives, medical directors, directors of managed care, planners, and administrators will all benefit from the book's focus on case management as an overall patient care strategy.

Catalog No. E99-027102 (must be included when ordering)
1995. 160 pages, 22 figures, 4 appendixes, index.
$52.00 (AHA members, $42.00)

Outpatient Case Management: Strategies for a New Reality
edited by Michelle Regan Donovan and Theodore A. Matson

Outpatient Case Management presents a framework for implementing case management strategies in the outpatient arena. This book provides general guidelines on case management and underscores the importance of this tool in a changing health care delivery system. In-depth discussions cover: the planning agenda, needs assessment, and other special considerations for developing case management programs; building strong working relationships with private payers; creating a seamless continuum of care, comprehensive care planning, and communications between inpatient and outpatient service providers; and the role and function of the case manager, including cost control responsibilities.

Catalog No. E99-027100 (must be included when ordering)
1994. 298 pages, 20 figures, 8 tables.
$58.95 (AHA members, $48.95)

Calculated Risk: A Provider's Guide to Assessing and Controlling the Financial Risk of Managed Care
Edited by Bruce S. Pyenson, FSA, MAAA
Milliman & Robertson, Inc.

This book presents the strategies and tools to help you analyze your current business and determine what needs to change to assume the various forms of managed care risk, including capitation. You'll benefit from experience-tested approaches, including the applications of actuarial cost models from the nation's foremost actuarial and consulting firm, Milliman & Robertson, Inc.

Catalog No. E99-131001 (must be included when ordering)
1995. 7880 pages, 19 figures, bibliography.
$32.00 (AHA members, $25.00)

To order, call TOLL FREE
1-800-AHA-2626